YOGA
for
pregnancy

Wendy Teasdill

Foreword by Michel Odent

Gaia Books Limited

For Iona, Eleanor and Belinda

A GAIA ORIGINAL

Books from Gaia celebrate the vision of Gaia, the self-sustaining living Earth, and seek to help its readers live in greater personal and planetary harmony.

Editor	Sarah Chapman
Designer	Sarah Theodosiou
Illustrator	Lucy Su
Photographer	Steve Teague
Managing Editor	Pip Morgan
Production	Lyn Kirby
Direction	Lucy Guenot, Patrick Nugent

Registered Trade Mark of Gaia Books Limited

First published in the United Kingdom in 2000 by
Gaia Books Ltd, 66 Charlotte Street, London W1P 1LR
and 20 High Street, Stroud, Gloucestershire GL5 1AZ

ISBN 1-85675-165-1

A catalogue record of this book is available from the British Library.

Printed and bound by Kyodo, Singapore

10 9 8 7 6 5 4 3 2 1

Publisher's note

YOGA
for
pregnancy

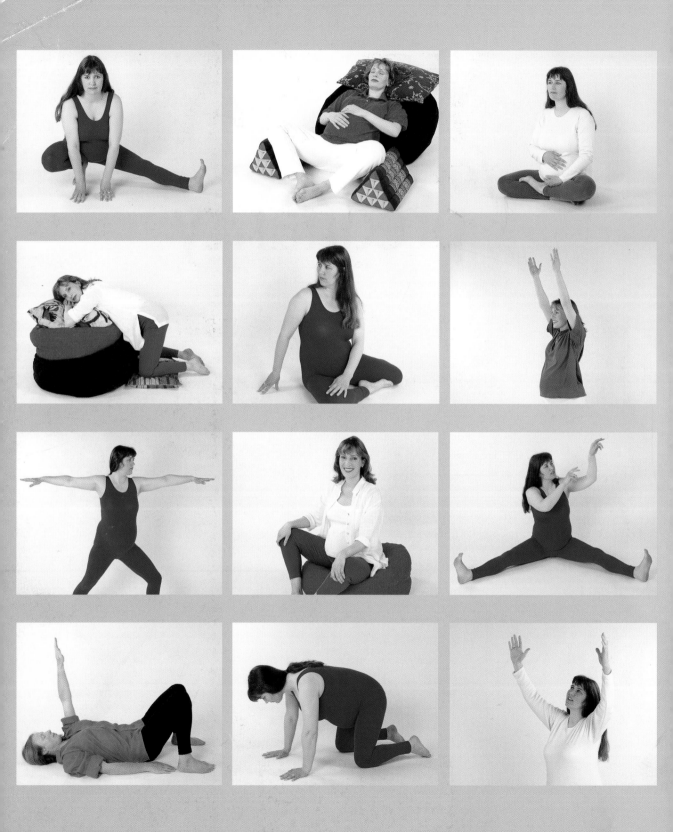

Contents

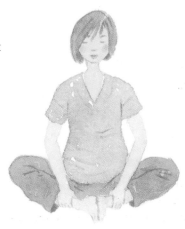

Foreword

We must pay tribute to Wendy Teasdill for sharing her holistic approach to life with mothers-to-be. Today one cannot imagine a more vital topic than the well-being of unborn children. At the Primal Health Research Centre we have been exploring the correlation between the 'primal period' (that includes foetal life) and later health and behaviour. *Yoga for Pregnancy* is published at the very time when scientific researchers are suddenly 'discovering' the concept of the uterine environment. During the 1990s a huge number of studies have suggested that the quality of our life in the womb determines to a great extent our future well-being. In the light of what we now know, we must radically revise our understanding of health and disease.

This aspect of the scientific revolution has many practical implications. One of them is a renewed interest in the work of those who try, like Wendy, to influence in a positive way the emotional states of pregnant women. These in turn can affect the growth and development of the baby in the womb. For example, an unhappy emotional state in the mother is associated with a high level of the hormone cortisol, which tends to restrict foetal growth. This book will help women recover a better hormonal balance during pregnancy.

Yoga for Pregnancy will also help readers realize that nutrition is an integral part of a yogic lifestyle. Yogic dietary principles are perfectly in accordance with the recommendations dictated by a modern scientific approach, with its emphasis on eating the less polluted foods at the beginning of the food chain.

I usually claim that pregnant women should not read books about pregnancy and birth. Their time is too precious. They should, rather, watch the moon and sing to their baby in the womb. *Yoga for Pregnancy* is an exception. In an ideal world, this book should be in the hands of all women who have not yet conceived a baby.

Dr Michel Odent, Head of Research,
The Primal Health Research Centre, London

Preface by Wendy Teasdill

Before I became pregnant I had been practising Iyengar yoga for 13 years; I was fit, energetic, and full of vitality. I assumed, like many women, that an expectant mother could simply adapt the traditional practice of yoga slightly. In the event of my own first pregnancy, though, yoga such as I was used to was suddenly out of the question. I fell victim to a paralyzing fatigue, accompanied by nausea and a tendency to vomit at the slightest exertion. Later in the pregnancy the baby's head pressed down on the sciatic nerve, and I could barely walk.

Nevertheless, I could not give up yoga. During those nine months I gradually learnt to adapt my practice as I went about finding out everything I could about yoga for pregnancy. I discovered a great deal of conflicting and confusing advice, and my only true yardstick was my own body, with which I felt more in tune – despite, or perhaps because of, the unexpected limitations – than ever before.

During my pregnancy I intuitively chose slow and gentle movements, modifying everything I did and sinking into a meditative state as I discovered the most effective positions. At the same time I began teaching yoga to pregnant women, which also raised many questions. As I gradually found out the answers to these, I incorporated them into the yoga sessions. My second pregnancy was quite different from the first, and though I still practised the gentler approach I had developed previously, I found that I could now include more active poses with ease. Grateful for the wider experience, I broadened the scope of my pregnancy yoga teaching.

As I write, I am in my third pregnancy, a series of swings between the fragile and the energetic sensations of the previous two. The seemingly perverse fluctuations of pregnancy remind me of the enormous versatility of yoga: within a framework of certain ground rules, there is no one set way to approach your practice during pregnancy.

This book is based not only upon my own experiences, but also upon those of the many women I have been lucky enough to teach. My aim is to present a wide range of yoga poses and their modifications, accompanied by clear guidance as to their suitability for varying levels of experience as well as for the different physical, mental and emotional states of pregnancy. My wish is that every woman may enjoy the gifts of yoga according to her individual needs during the nine sacred months of gestation and beyond.

Introduction

Yoga is an ancient and holistic system of harmonizing body, heart and mind. Pregnancy is a time of transition, when all manner of new sensations and experiences may arise. Yoga, when practised during pregnancy, will help you not only maintain your health and well-being but also bring peace and freedom to the body, heart and mind of both you and your child.

'Yoga' means 'union', and was originally developed several thousand years ago by hermits high up in the north of India (now Pakistan) as a means of stilling the mind. It consists of various exercises that are mostly based on animal movements. The movements are done slowly and meditatively, and combined with breath awareness. Yoga tones the muscles without straining them, promotes healthy blood flow, combats fatigue, balances the neuro-endocrine system, stabilizes emotions, reduces stress and reconciles all contradictions. Thus the physical body is flexed and strengthened in order to sit still, enabling us to explore the deeper reaches of meditation. In the process, the mind does indeed also become still.

Civilization has changed vastly since the dawn of yoga, but women give birth now just as they did then. Yoga brings us back to our instinctive, natural selves, making it possibly more vital to us today than it was to the forest-dwellers of old. The adaptibility of yoga means that it is an ideal form of exercise during the many changes of pregnancy. Appropriately taught and practised, it is an excellent way of preparing for the birth of a baby.

The practice of yoga during pregnancy can do much to improve and maintain health and well-being. It will boost your energy and refresh you when you feel fatigued, and it will also calm you if you are over-active, helping you sleep more soundly. Gentle stretching will counter-

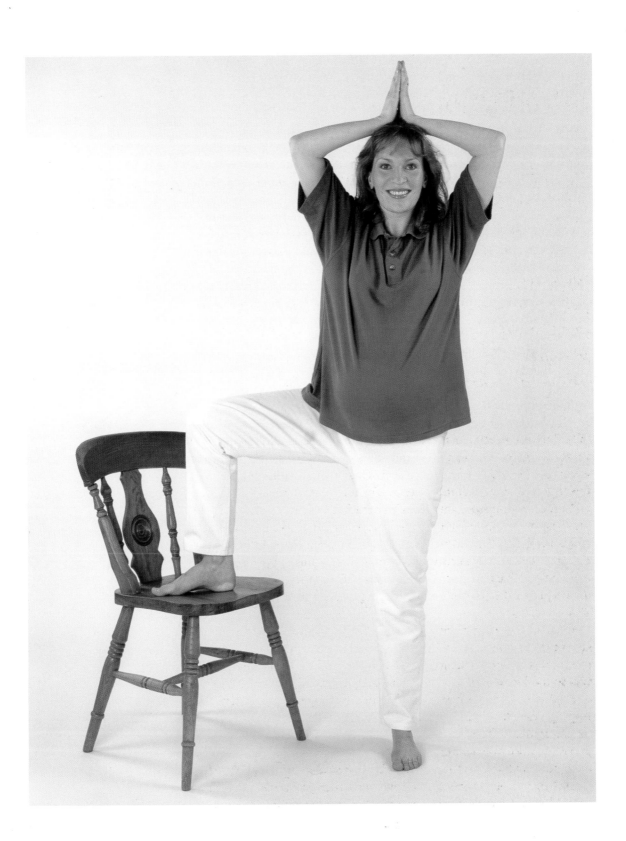

act tiredness, and tone the muscles without straining them. Yoga stimulates the relaxation response, removing the heavy feeling of fatigue and replacing it with nature's own light, 'feel-good' hormones, which help the body work at maximum efficiency.

Although regular yoga sessions won't guarantee a quick and easy delivery, you will find that if you are already used to doing yoga it will come into its own during childbirth. You will be able to accept whatever happens, trust your own instincts and 'go with' the experience of the contractions calmly. Tension is inimical to a smooth labour, and yoga allows your body to release tension, and to relax in harmony with the downward pull of gravity so that labour can progress without resistance. If the birth does not go according to plan, and you find yourself in a more challenging situation, you will be flexible enough to adapt without losing self-confidence. Women who have taken responsibility for their own health through yoga practice during pregnancy find that they heal more quickly and are less prone to postnatal depression than those who don't.

Yoga helps you build a harmonious bridge of contact with your baby within you. If you can bond with your child before he or she is born, this will help ease the transition from foetus to baby, from gestation to birth, from pregnancy to motherhood. Even if the first days of the new baby's life leave you no time to practise, they will be easier if you have done yoga during pregnancy. Yoga not only reveals the transformative powers of pregnancy but is the catalyst by which we may build a firmer, happier and healthier future for our children – from within.

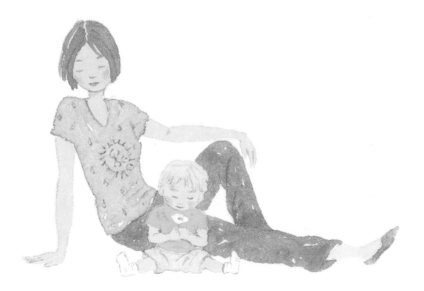

Part One

Your well-being during pregnancy

'Living in accordance with natural hierarchy is not a matter of following a series of rigid rules or structuring your days with lifeless commandments or codes of conduct. The world has order and power and richness that can teach you how to conduct your life artfully, with kindness to others and care for yourself.'

Chogyam Trungpa, from *Shambhala, The Sacred Path of the Warrior*

CHAPTER ONE

How yoga enhances pregnancy

By practising yoga, an expectant mother invites harmony into her body. Since the baby within is not only dependent on you physically but also sensitive to your mental and emotional states, equilibrium can only enhance the mother–baby bond. The baby feels more secure and your confidence in your innate capabilities increases.

Pregnancy has a profound impact on the body. Whether you know from the moment of conception that you are pregnant, or take months to realize it, you are undergoing great physical changes. Hormones are invading the system at a hundred times their usual rate, affecting all areas of your being. At first these changes are not visible. You may simply feel below par, but your body is working to maximum capacity. The digestive system, for example, slows down and may seem sluggish, but it extracts and processes the goodness from food much more efficiently than usual.

Pregnancy is also a time of great emotional adjustment, as you prepare for the challenges of birth and parenthood. You may feel happy and excited if the pregnancy was anticipated; if it was unplanned you may feel shock and apprehension, and coming to terms with the pregnancy may take time. No matter how pleased you are to be pregnant, however, you will probably find that at first your emotions are closer to the surface than usual, and that you have less control over them.

The nine months of pregnancy are divided into three three-monthly periods, or 'trimesters', each of which brings its own changes and adjustments to be made. Some people even refer to 'the fourth trimester' – that is, the first three months of the baby's life.

The first trimester is the period of greatest physical adaptation. The blood pressure drops and the breasts swell and feel tender. Nausea and fatigue, vomiting, mood swings, irritability, lack of appetite, constipation, dizziness, headaches and shortness of breath are all possible side-effects

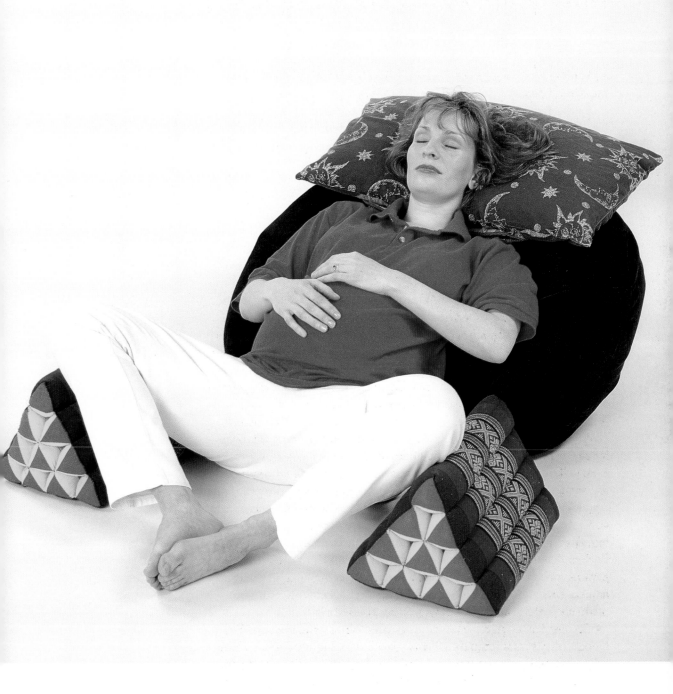

of the raised hormone levels. Regular yoga practice will help temper these symptoms, and learning breath awareness and relaxation techniques will increase your energy.

All these imbalances are temporary, and the body usually stabilizes by the second trimester. This is often referred to as 'the blooming period' in which energy returns, the hair shines and the skin glows, and the full, positive effects of pregnancy can be experienced. Traditional yoga positions must be adapted to conform to your changing shape and weight, but a wide range of poses is possible.

By the end of the pregnancy you may feel invaded from within, pushed to the far peripheries of the bulge that dominates your every movement. Yet with a little gentle stretching and an increased emphasis on breathing exercises and meditation, it is easy to remember that you are still capable of self-determination.

Body awareness

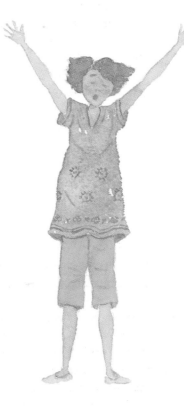

During pregnancy, as the uterus expands and grows heavier with the increasing weight of the baby, the body's centre of gravity alters and encourages the lumbar spine to arch. This may cause the shoulders to hunch in compensation, which in turn may cause severe aching in the lower back and neck. Yoga teaches body awareness, by showing you your areas of tension and imbalance, and by increasing suppleness and the ability to relax. Developing body awareness is not just confined to the time we spend doing yoga, but benefits every aspect of our lives. All daily activities, if done thoughtfully, can enhance our physical well-being during pregnancy.

It is not only by moving into certain positions, called asanas, that yoga facilitates body awareness. Breathing is an integral part of yoga, and no movement is done without appropriate breath co-ordination. Though simple techniques are used, they are enormously effective. The synchronized stretching and breathing of yoga relieve bad posture, poor circulation and sluggishness, which can combine to form a build-up of toxins in the body. The exercises open up trouble spots such as the lumbar spine, shoulders, neck and backs of the knees, and the enhanced flow of oxygen-rich blood flushes out toxins.

As the volume of blood in your body increases so much in pregnancy, it is especially important to encourage healthy blood flow. This generates a clear, buoyant feeling, however big your bump is. Improved circulation also acts upon the endocrine system, encouraging glands to work more efficiently. In addition, women whose skins are used to stretching with yoga rarely get stretch marks during pregnancy.

Once you have become used to putting your body into certain positions, during labour these positions will come easily and naturally. Likewise, if you are familiar with breathing exercises, efficient breathing during childbirth will come of its own accord.

The mind and emotions

As well as optimizing physical health, the practice of yoga during pregnancy calms the mind. The apparent turmoil into which the body is thrown can create corresponding emotional and mental turbulence. The yogic fusion of slow, meditative movements and breath awareness brings clarity and confidence to an indecisive mind and contentment instead of worry.

The combination of pregnancy hormones with yoga breathing exercises may, however, bring long-buried emotions to the surface (often to do with the relationship with one's own mother). If this happens, it is best to let the feelings arise naturally in the controlled environment of yoga practice. Tears and grief may appear for no apparent reason, but it is better to weep than to push the feelings down again. If repressed, the emotions will only reappear. By allowing them expression, release and freedom will follow, which in turn will ease delivery and lighten your relationship with your child.

The inner security that you will achieve from yoga prepares you for the birth experience by giving you the resources on which to draw when in childbirth. Having benefited from yoga during pregnancy, in labour you will find it easier to withdraw from the outer world of distractions to the instinctive realm within. Because you have developed flexibility of mind as well as body, you will find it easier to accept and adapt to whatever happens when the time comes to deliver.

The first trimester

The first trimester (or three-monthly period) of the 40 weeks of pregnancy officially begins two weeks before you conceive – that is, on the first day of your last period, if your menstrual cycle is regular – and continues until about 12 to 14 weeks. The time of fertilization is counted as the end of the second week.

After conception, the secretion of two hormones, progesterone and oestrogen, increases dramatically and suppresses menstruation, allowing the fertilized egg to embed itself in the wall of the uterus. These hormones help the body adapt to the pregnancy, and will be produced in great quantities until the baby is born. They are produced by the

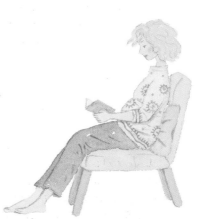

corpus luteum, a gland on the ovary, until about the 13th week, when the placenta is sufficiently developed to take over their manufacture. Progesterone and oestrogen relax and soften the ligaments and organs to accommodate the growing baby and in preparation for the birth. They also cause the breasts to swell in readiness for eventual breast-feeding. These and other hormones are responsible for the side-effects of the first trimester such as mood swings, nausea and fatigue.

Mood swings

For the first few weeks of pregnancy the presence of extra hormones may not be obvious and you may feel much as normal. It is at about the sixth week, as the head, heart, circulation and spine of the embryo are forming, that the flood of hormones becomes noticeable. You may accommodate them easily, or be overwhelmed by them. Even if you are a normally capable bundle of energy, you may find yourself dissolving in tears unexpectedly, or feel that you are going through a personality crisis (which of course you are). Yet this is a positive and not a negative transition, preparing you for the great changes ahead. Perhaps the greater the apparent crisis, the more sensitive you will be as a mother. Yoga, with its emphasis on breathing, can help you reassert a certain amount of calm objectivity to carry you through the changes.

Nausea

The nausea and sickness common during the first three or four months are often called 'morning sickness' but can occur at any time of day. It is worth trying the various possible remedies to find one that works for you.

Low blood sugar levels may aggravate nausea, and can be raised by eating little and often. Fruit is especially good, since fructose (fruit sugar) is quickly absorbed into the blood. Don't get up in the morning until you have eaten a dry biscuit with a cup of hot sweet tea. If you find tea unpalatable, try a glass of milk, or peppermint or ginger tea.

Deficiency of the Vitamin B complex may cause nausea. Vitamin B6, found in bananas, raspberry leaf, basil, ginger and peppermint tea, will help relieve the condition.

Zinc deficiency may also be a cause of nausea, according to recent research. Since red meat is a major source of zinc, vegetarians may either take a zinc supplement or try eating plenty of pumpkin seeds, maize and green vegetables.

Bending over from the waist may provoke nausea at any time because it will irritate the vagus nerve, which is connected to the stom-

Caution: It is important to realize the difference between the normal discomforts of pregnancy and a genuine medical condition. If you have any worries, seek medical advice. Certain conditions, including high blood pressure, diabetes, vaginal bleeding, acute dizziness, headaches, shortness of breath, placenta praevia and pre-eclampsia, need medical supervision.

A healthy woman who takes charge of her own well-being during pregnancy – by practising yoga, eating sensibly, being aware of her movements in daily life and resting when necessary – will cut down the need for medical intervention enormously.

ach and controls digestive activity. This nerve is especially sensitive during pregnancy. To avoid discomfort, squat down instead of bending to pick things up. Squatting also exercises the legs, opens the pelvis and stretches the lower back.

Fatigue

Chronic, sometimes overwhelming, fatigue is common during the first three months, when the embryo is attaching itself to the lining of the uterine cavity. Fatigue is the body's way of telling you to take care of the pregnancy by resting as much as you can. Don't do any jumping or lifting, or any yoga exercises except for those described in chapter 3.

Low blood pressure

The drop in blood pressure during early pregnancy can result in light-headedness. Avoid standing still for any length of time because there is a risk of fainting, especially if you have not eaten. When doing forward bends, either standing or sitting, don't hang your head down. (This applies throughout pregnancy, though the reasons for this will change.)

Relaxation of involuntary muscles

The hormonal flood causes all the involuntary muscles to relax. These are the smooth muscles lining the intestines, the blood and lymph vessels, and the bladder and the uterus itself. During the first trimester the uterus is still in the pelvis, pressing on the bladder, and this, together with the relaxation effect, means you might need to empty your bladder more often than usual. Urinary infections are also more likely. Drinking cranberry juice is helpful, and the Tailor's pose, Baddha Konasana (page 60), is invaluable.

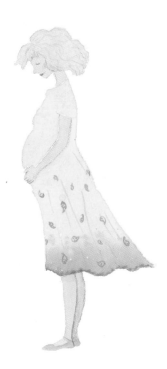

Digestion takes longer and you may become constipated. Drinking enough fluids and eating plenty of fruit and other fibre-rich foods will bring some relief, and so will yoga. After the first trimester, gentle twists and forward bends stimulate the colon into action.

As the walls of the blood vessels soften, pockets of blood can accumulate, possibly resulting in varicose veins and haemorrhoids. Don't cross your legs while sitting, don't stand too long in one spot, and elevate the legs as much as possible. All yoga, including breathing exercises, will encourage the blood to flow more freely.

Mucous membranes can become congested. Usually the nostrils block alternately. If you lie on your side with the blocked nostril uppermost, it will soon clear, or you could try Neti (page 110).

The second trimester

Sometime between the 11th and 13th week of pregnancy, the corpus luteum in the ovary shrinks and the placenta takes over progesterone production. This transition into the second trimester can sometimes cause pain similar to menstrual cramps for a few days. Miscarriages are commoner at this time than at any other, so take extra care now to listen to your body and not do anything too strenuous. Relaxing postures such as the supported Corpse pose, Savasana (see page 44), and the supported reclining Thunderbolt, Supta Virasana (see page 104), are most suitable.

This is often the happiest and most comfortable stage of pregnancy. The pregnancy is well established, the placenta is making its own progesterone and hormone levels balance out, bringing greater stability of mind and body. Nausea and fatigue typically – though not always – disappear, the breasts remain the same size for the next three months, and the appetite returns.

Foetal growth is rapid, and by the 14th week the heart, brain, lungs, kidneys and other organs are formed. The baby's heart – beating about twice as fast as your own – can be heard with a hand-held electronic monitor. By about the 18th to 20th week in a first pregnancy, and a month or so earlier in subsequent ones, you will feel the first foetal movements. At first they produce a vague sensation, like butterflies or fish, and gradually become more definite as the baby grows and moves and kicks more vigorously.

The uterus has enlarged out of the pelvis up into the abdomen, and will continue to grow up towards the ribcage, relieving pressure on the bladder. An increase in skin pigmentation may cause darkening of the nipples and a dark line known as the linea nigra from the navel to the pubic area. A 'mask' of darker skin may develop on the face, and you may also notice a darkening of freckles and moles. Since you are now making a third more blood than usual, the heart grows accordingly and must work harder, and you will want to drink more.

Exercise and movement

Blood pressure should return to normal, and any dizziness should disappear. A wide range of yoga poses can be done easily, although some may be uncomfortable unless you modify them. Many of the poses will counteract discomforts such as backache, now more likely as the increasing weight of the uterus stresses the lower back. Standing poses against a wall or door, perhaps using a chair, as well as an all-fours pose

Miscarriage

Most miscarriages occur in the first 12 weeks. If you have a tendency to miscarry, or have reason to believe that you might be susceptible, avoid standing poses and twists altogether. It is beneficial to do forward bends after the first trimester, and sitting and supine poses are also good, since they increase blood flow to the uterine area and stimulate foetal growth.

If you are in any doubt about a pose, don't do it. Should a miscarriage threaten, the only suitable pose is the Corpse (Savasana).

such as the Cat and its variations, squats, forward bends and gentle twists, are all helpful.

When resting or sleeping, facilitate blood flow either by lying on your side, supporting your upper knee with cushions, or, if you prefer to be supine, by elevating the back and head. Another alternative is to lie flat on your back and bend the knees, planting the feet firmly on the floor by the buttocks.

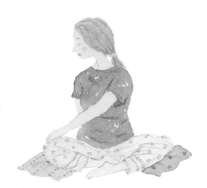

Care of ligaments and tendons

The hormone relaxin, secreted by the placenta, softens the ligaments that join bone to bone around the joints, and the tendons that attach muscle to bone. If you already practise yoga, you may find some poses easier than before, and beginners may find yoga easier than they had imagined. Overstretching can be dangerous, however, because stretched ligaments and tendons, unlike muscles, will not revert to their original size. Loose ligaments result in loose joints, which in turn cause uneven wearing of cartilage, possibly leading to problems later in life. This especially applies to the sacro-iliac joint, where the lumbar spine joins the pelvis, as there are no muscles to counteract the effects of over-stretched ligaments. Even if you find that you can stretch further forward than before, don't be tempted. Simply enjoy the ease with which you can sink into poses within your normal capabilities.

The third trimester

The third trimester is the period between 28 and 40 weeks. After the 28th week the foetus becomes viable, that is, theoretically capable of surviving outside the womb. Most babies born after 32 weeks survive, since their lungs are now mature enough to breathe.

You will feel a variety of strong movements as your baby kicks and rolls from side to side, especially when you are resting. The baby's body grows more in proportion to the head, and fat is deposited under the skin. By the eighth month the uterus fills the abdominal cavity, causing pressure on your stomach and lungs.

The baby will engage its head in the pelvis, ready for birth, any time from now on in a first pregnancy. In subsequent pregnancies, because the uterus is more stretched and there is more room, the head may not engage until labour starts. When the head goes down you may feel your uterus drop. This 'lightening' takes some of the pressure off the lungs, making breathing easier. Pressure on the bladder increases, how-ever, and the frequent need to urinate may disrupt sleep.

Endorphins
Endorphins are natural opiates secreted by the brain to counteract pain and create a feeling of well-being. Throughout pregnancy their production is higher than usual, which perhaps accounts for the 'pregnancy glow'. They increase when you do physical exercise, including yoga, and when you are relaxed. Even more are released during labour, in order to help you cope with the contractions.

The ligaments of the pelvis soften further, and you may experience discomfort in the pelvic joints. As the pelvis continues to expand in preparation for the birth, the joints at the front and back of the pelvis may loosen enough to cause aching and even trap a nerve so that walking and sitting become restricted. Yoga poses to relieve the pressure include squatting, the Cat, the Child, the Sphinx and the Tailor's pose, done sitting on a rolled blanket. All these positions can be done for extended lengths of time. It is also pleasant to lie on the back with the legs up against a wall, either together or outstretched, but only if it does not make you breathless or cause tingling toes.

According to Ayurvedic medicine, the traditional science of Indian healing, it is during the last eight weeks of gestation that the mother transfers a vital energy known as 'Ojas' to the baby. Ojas is an essential component of all the bodily tissues; combined with prana, the life force, it is responsible for hormonal balance, the auto-immune system and intelligence. Babies born before 32 weeks are denied this essence and it is to this, rather than the fact the lungs are not sufficiently developed, that their lower chances of survival are attributed. Ojas is also believed to be present in the mother's milk.

The final month

During the last month or so before the birth, the greatly enlarged uterus makes movement cumbersome, and pressure on the stomach may cause heartburn and even vomiting. To ease the problem, eat smaller amounts more frequently, avoid fatty and spicy foods, don't eat just before going to bed and prop yourself up on several pillows to sleep. Drinking mint tea or milk may help.

As the continually enlarging abdomen pulls on the lumbar vertebral muscles, neither standing nor sitting in a conventional position will be comfortable. Older women, who have never done yoga as such, may tell you that all they wanted to do in the last month of pregnancy was go down on their hands and knees and scrub the floor. This position is like the Cat, which is a most helpful pose at this stage.

Because your heart's output has increased and because of the pressure from the enlarged uterus on the lungs, you will experience breathlessness. To relieve this, reduce pressure on the lower ribs by squatting rather than bending forward when doing daily tasks, and open the shoulders and straighten the lumbar spine whenever you can. Doing a supported seated angle pose such as Upavista Konasana (see page 117) will create more room in the upper abdomen for both

The pelvic floor
Throughout pregnancy, the strain on the pelvic floor – the group of muscles at the base of the body – will intensify. The pelvic floor supports the weight of the internal organs, and during the last weeks of pregnancy this can be considerable. If the pelvic floor is not toned, the reduced elasticity may prolong labour and cause incontinence, both before and after the birth. Many yoga positions in themselves serve to strengthen this area, and there are specific pelvic floor exercises (see pages 46–7) that cannot be begun too soon.

digestion and breathing, and will help increase your energy levels.

Towards the end of the final month you may begin to feel as if the pregnancy is going to last for ever, and lassitude can be a problem. Rather than give in to lethargy, however, take the increased difficulty of movement as a signal to turn your attention inward. Focus on breath awareness and breath control as you emphasize the slower, more meditative poses in your practice. Concentrate also on visualizations for the birth, relaxation in the Corpse pose and meditation (see chapter 5).

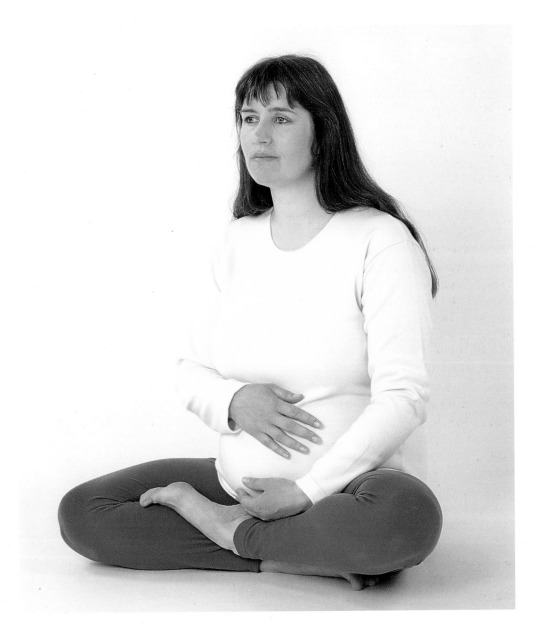

CHAPTER TWO

Yoga in everyday life

Yoga's holistic approach to life has special value during pregnancy. Through co-ordinated stretching and simple breathing exercises, the body is at once strengthened and relaxed while the mind is calmed. The yogic diet will also benefit you and your baby, bringing health and vitality and helping you towards the best possible pregnancy and delivery.

Because yoga is so good at combating stress, it is perhaps even more relevant in today's hectic society than it was in earlier times. Yoga helps the endocrine system function more efficiently, boosts the immune system, balances the emotions and gives you a feeling of well-being. Yoga enables us to live more clearly and peacefully in the present moment.

Diet is an integral part of the yogic way of life. The yogic diet is nourishing and well balanced, based on natural foods such as fruit, grains and vegetables. Full of prana, the life force, it keeps the body lean and supple and the mind clear, making it most suitable for the practice of yoga. It is also the ideal diet for your unborn baby, since it offers the most goodness and the fewest toxins.

In yogic philosophy all life is sacred, and it is impossible to contemplate eating meat or fish. If you are not a vegetarian already, however, pregnancy is no time in which to become one. But you might find that yoga practice makes you more aware of what you eat and of the different effects different foods have on you.

Although after the first trimester you can practise yoga in a daily session, as a sequence of poses like those described in chapter 4, the poses can also be done one at a time, woven into your daily life during normal activities whenever you have a spare moment. They can be used to enhance ordinary movements such as standing, sitting and walking. In this way yoga will help relieve aches and pains such as backache, and will also increase your suppleness, help strengthen your legs and loosen your hip joints in preparation for the birth itself.

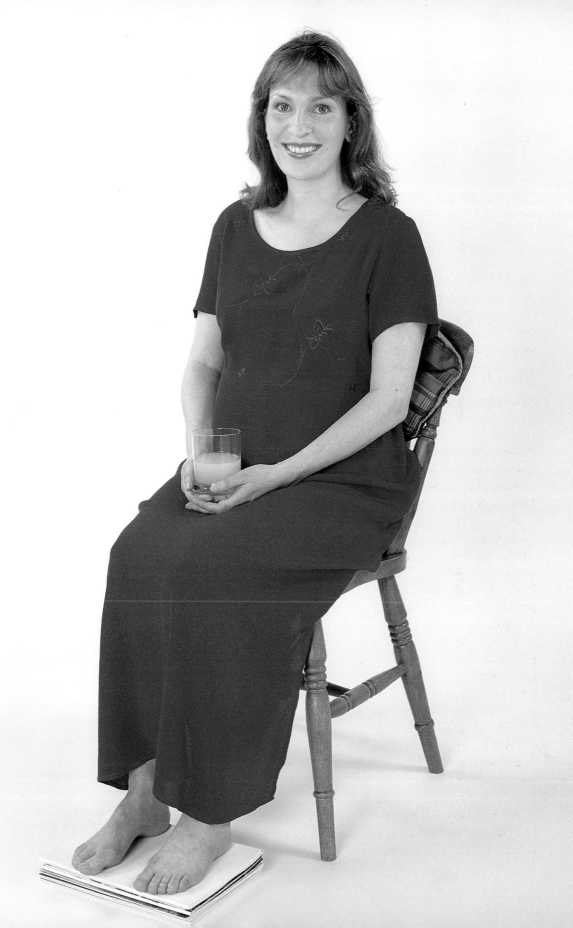

Your daily practice

Ideally, practise yoga in a clean cool place, away from direct sunlight and wind, free of insects, noise and other intrusions. If possible, have a space reserved only for yoga; if not, you can quickly create your 'space apart' by putting down a mat or a rug.

Any time is a good time for yoga, except just after a meal. Even then, however, you can sit in certain poses, such as the Tailor's pose page 60, which aids digestion and widens the pelvis. The best time to practise yoga is first thing in the morning, when your mind is at its clearest, but if you find that nausea makes this impossible, two hours after a meal is also suitable. If you leave it too long you may become nauseous or light-headed again. So plan ahead. By the evening, your body is more flexible and your mind more active, and yoga at that time will calm the mind and counteract insomnia, especially during the last trimester.

You are the best judge of how much yoga to do at any given time, and you will probably feel quite different during each trimester. Match your practice to how you feel – for example, if you feel tired, don't wear yourself out with warrior poses, but concentrate on sitting and breathing. Even if you feel lively, counteract active poses with restful ones, and always end with relaxation in the Corpse pose, even if you only have a few minutes. And stop when you have had enough. Several 15- or 20-minute sessions a day, which revive you, are more beneficial than an hour-long session that tires you out.

Throughout pregnancy and during the postpartum period, practise yoga gently. Strenuous exercise produces adrenaline, which blocks the body's ability to produce natural relaxants. Too much vigour may also result in aching muscles or nausea.

Caution: Throughout pregnancy, the following poses are contra-indicated

- double leg-lifts

- cross-over and reversed poses (except for the reverse triangle, which can be done in a modified form)

- back bends (these put too much pressure on the already stressed and softened ligaments of the lumbar spine)

- positions that involve lying on your front, for example the Cobra

- inverted poses and shoulder stands (see page 50)

- any position that doesn't feel right

Guidelines for practice

- Wear loose, comfortable clothing.
- Practise in bare feet unless it is cold.
- Practise somewhere quiet and out of the sun.
- Don't practise directly after a meal – wait one or two hours, depending on how much you've eaten.
- Modify the postures according to your development, trimester, experience and inclination.
- Don't over-exert yourself, hold standing poses for too long or prolong a yoga session so that you become tired. Balance active poses with restful ones according to how you feel.
- If you are experienced in yoga you can adapt most of the postures you are used to, with the exception of the few listed above, right. If you are a beginner don't be too ambitious.
- Listen to your body. It is your best guide.

Yoga in daily activities

Yoga is not just to be done in a session, separate from the rest of your life, but something you can integrate into all your daily activities. Swimming and walking, for example, if done with awareness, are similar to yoga, since they combine movement with rhythmic breathing. If you invite it, yoga can be a constant companion in your life.

Standing

When pregnant, you may feel light-headed if you stand for too long in one place. During the first trimester this is because your blood pressure is lower than normal; later in the pregnancy it may be because the weight of the uterus restricts the blood return from the legs (which also provokes varicose veins). When preparing food or doing other tasks usually performed while standing, try to do them sitting down at a table or, even better, sitting or squatting on the floor. When you have to be standing up, for washing up, say, use a footstool and rest your feet on it at alternate intervals.

When you do stand, be aware of your stance and try not to let the small of your back give in to the increasing weight of the abdomen by arching. Instead, use the Mountain pose (see page 53): tuck your tailbone under and allow your legs and pelvis to take the weight of the abdomen. Regular practice of this in yoga sessions will help it come to you more easily even when standing in supermarket queues. Correct posture will prevent the abdominal muscles from sagging and counteract low back pain, stiff shoulders and headaches.

Walking

You can adapt the Mountain pose to walking. If you develop a sense of your central axis during the first trimester or before, this can stay with you, bestowing inner poise and outer stability. During the last trimester, you may experience difficulty in walking, however much yoga you do, as the baby's head engages in the cervix (at about the 32nd week in a first pregnancy, but often not until labour starts during subsequent ones). The baby's head may also press on your bladder and possibly on nerves in the area. To counteract these problems, go down on your hands and knees in the Cat pose, or rest on your forearms, so that your pelvis is higher than your shoulders, in the Sphinx. Of course, this is easy to do at home, but may prove difficult if you are out. A forward bend is socially acceptable and you can do it against any convenient chair-back or window-ledge.

Bending and lifting

If you can delegate, do so. If you must lift a heavy weight, such as a child, face it square on, bend your knees and, with your feet fairly wide apart and slightly turned out, squat down. Bend forward from the hips. As you lift, hold the object or child close to your body and use your thigh muscles to push yourself up. Keep your weight over your heels, and don't twist your back as you lift. When changing direction, turn your feet first and then your body, not vice versa.

If possible, don't reach up to lift things from a height. This can cause the back to arch, and the extra weight of the uterus can compress the spine. If you cannot avoid lifting from a height, do a pelvic tilt first, keep your back as straight as you can and use your arm muscles to take the weight.

Carrying

Carrying heavy weights may easily distend the ligaments supporting the uterus and cause back pain. If you must carry anything, either use a backpack or distribute the weight evenly. Carry a small child on alternate hips, and keep your spine upright.

Sitting

Sitting in a deep low armchair allows the spine to sag and the vertebrae to compress, causing backache. Always use a chair that supports the spine well, and that also allows you to tilt the pelvis and to place your feet flat upon the floor. Put your feet on books or a footstool if they don't reach the floor.

Sitting on a chair with your legs crossed at the thigh will constrict blood flow, causing or exacerbating varicose veins. Sitting cross-legged on the floor, however, or with the soles of the feet together, is most beneficial, since this position allows the pelvis to widen, and stretches both the pelvic floor and the inner thigh muscles. As your pregnancy advances, sitting on a low stool, cushion or beanbag will allow the same opening while giving space to your growing uterus.

Squatting or sitting on a low stool during pregnancy has many other benefits. While stretching the pelvic floor and inner thigh muscles, it also elongates the vertebrae of the lower back, reducing strain on the spine, and strengthens the ankles. This position encourages your baby to get into a good position for the birth, and gives you increased strength and suppleness, improving your well-being during pregnancy and your ability to withstand the rigours of labour.

Caution: If your baby is in the breech (head up) position, don't squat during the last eight weeks.

Lying down and getting up

When lying down, do so in stages, as it is important not to strain the abdominal muscles.

• First, step forward and kneel on one knee, then on both knees.
• Place your hands on the floor and support your weight as you bring your hips to the floor on the side that is comfortable for you, and sit down.
• Bring your elbow to the floor on the side you have chosen; lean on your elbow and lie down on your side.
• Roll from your side on to your back if you wish (caution: see below).
• To get up from a supine position, roll on to your side and reverse the process. Go slowly, since to stand up too quickly may cause dizziness, especially first thing in the morning.
• When getting into bed, first sit down on the side of the bed; then lean sideways on your elbows and roll your knees up on to the bed.
• Reverse the process to stand up again, going slowly.

Resting and sleeping

As your baby grows, lying flat on your back will become increasingly uncomfortable and undesirable: the weight of the enlarged uterus presses down on the main veins returning from the legs, impeding blood flow to the baby. If you prefer sleeping on your back, support yourself as you would for relaxation in the Corpse pose, shown on pages 40 and 44. This relaxes the lumbar vertebrae, easing backache.

   Lying on your side is often the most comfortable resting and sleeping position, especially in mid- and late pregnancy. The left side is supposed to be more calming, but this will depend on how your baby is lying. Place a pillow or two under your head and another under the bent knee of the upper leg. This feels relaxing and avoids compressing the uterus. A smaller cushion or pad placed under your bump during late pregnancy will prevent strain on the abdominal muscles. Experiment to see what is most comfortable for you.

Caution: Don't lie flat on your back if you are uncomfortable: have the foot of your bed raised with blocks so that your legs are above your heart, especially if you are prone to varicose veins.

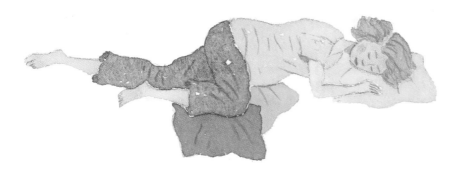

Going up and down stairs

This can be one of the most tiring mundane activities during pregnancy, but a little thought can turn it into a beneficial exercise. Place the whole foot on each stair, and deliberately relax your shoulders as you go. Go slowly, and breathe naturally in time with your steps.

Typing

Typing may not seem strenuous, but the repeated action of ligaments softened by pregnancy can cause permanent repetitive strain injury (RSI). Shoulders can, if unwatched, hunch forwards over the keyboard, causing tension. Take regular breaks from typing, and take any opportunity you can to raise your sternum up off your abdomen with a quick Cow-head pose (part 2; see page 93). Gently shake your wrists and do neck exercises regularly; stretch the lumbar spine as often as you can by doing a standing forward bend against the back of the chair.

Picking things up from the floor

You will soon find that bending to pick things up off the floor is uncomfortable: you compress your lungs and uterus, feel breathless, awkward and even sick. You can avoid this if you bend your knees and, keeping your back straight, squat. If you have to move about while on the floor, crawl around on all fours if need be.

Watching television

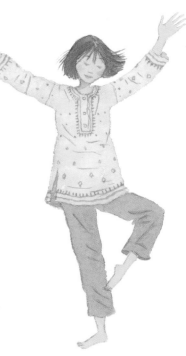

It is all too easy to want to slump in front of a television when pregnant, but since sitting in a deep armchair can cause or increase back pain, choose a more upright chair if possible and take care how you position yourself. Better still, sit on the floor in a symmetrical position with a cushion under the buttocks, so that you can then tilt your pelvis forward rather than back. You could also lean forward over a beanbag, as in the supported Child's pose (page 117), or sit upright on a straight-backed chair. If you can persuade your partner to massage your back at the same time, watching television can be a fruitful activity.

Dancing

Dancing with a pelvic focus can be very enjoyable while you are pregnant. Do pelvic circles and tilts, wave your arms freely, take small steps, and lose your weight in the music. Some women find that they enjoy dancing during the first stage of labour, since they find that the movements help ease the pain of contractions.

Relieving backache

Few women go through pregnancy without experiencing backache, especially during the third trimester. This is a time when the ligaments attaching the uterus to the spine are most stressed by the extra weight you are carrying. For this reason, avoid all positions that arch the back. Because your ligaments and tendons are soft as a result of hormonal changes, they can more easily be stretched out of shape, which can lead to permanent injury. Sometimes the baby's position – with its back to your back, for example – puts extra stress on your upper back, causing severe aching between the shoulder blades. Aches and pains of old injuries, which you thought had healed years ago, may, on account of this hormone-soaking, reappear. They will go away again once the baby is born.

Low back pain

The key to counteracting low back pain lies in remembering to tilt the pelvis every so often, so that the lower back flattens. Various exercises described in part 2, such as lunges and sitting against a wall, will help relieve low back pain, but you don't have to be in the middle of a yoga session to do them. You can choose any time and any convenient wall or tree. Do them at the beginning of a session, and in public – anyone seeing your condition will understand. You can also do them standing up in a swimming pool, which is especially relaxing since the water supports your weight. Take advantage of ledges and the backs of chairs to do a standing forward bend (see page 55).

Upper back pain

Pain in the upper back can be counteracted by upward and lateral stretches of the shoulders. Helpful poses for back pain include hanging from a belt over a door and giving yourself a top-to-toe stretch whenever you feel like it (see page 90), and the Cat pose (below and page 56).

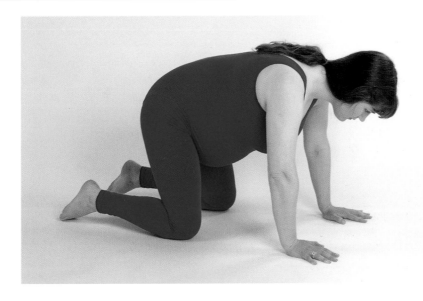

Working with the chakras

In the yogic tradition the chakras are seven energy centres arranged vertically up the spine, and linked to a different endocrine gland. Each chakra is represented by a lotus and associated with a colour. Chakras contain the essence of our conditioning and inform our personality, and are positively affected by yoga postures. Cultivating an intuitive awareness of the chakras during pregnancy can help shed inhibitions and release tension.

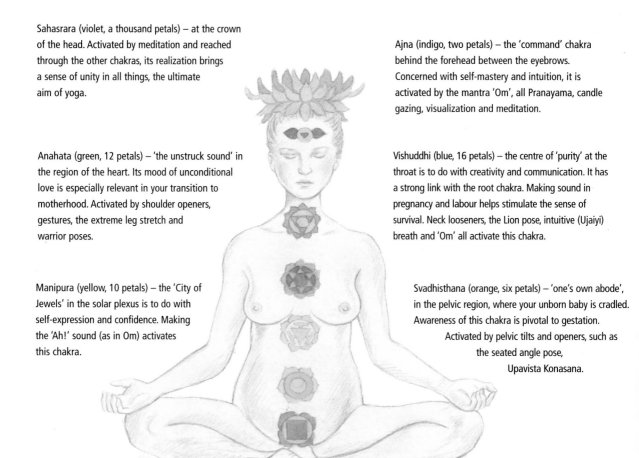

Sahasrara (violet, a thousand petals) – at the crown of the head. Activated by meditation and reached through the other chakras, its realization brings a sense of unity in all things, the ultimate aim of yoga.

Ajna (indigo, two petals) – the 'command' chakra behind the forehead between the eyebrows. Concerned with self-mastery and intuition, it is activated by the mantra 'Om', all Pranayama, candle gazing, visualization and meditation.

Anahata (green, 12 petals) – 'the unstruck sound' in the region of the heart. Its mood of unconditional love is especially relevant in your transition to motherhood. Activated by shoulder openers, gestures, the extreme leg stretch and warrior poses.

Vishuddhi (blue, 16 petals) – the centre of 'purity' at the throat is to do with creativity and communication. It has a strong link with the root chakra. Making sound in pregnancy and labour helps stimulate the sense of survival. Neck looseners, the Lion pose, intuitive (Ujaiyi) breath and 'Om' all activate this chakra.

Manipura (yellow, 10 petals) – the 'City of Jewels' in the solar plexus is to do with self-expression and confidence. Making the 'Ah!' sound (as in Om) activates this chakra.

Svadhisthana (orange, six petals) – 'one's own abode', in the pelvic region, where your unborn baby is cradled. Awareness of this chakra is pivotal to gestation. Activated by pelvic tilts and openers, such as the seated angle pose, Upavista Konasana.

Muladhara (red, four petals) – the 'root' chakra at the base of the body, including the cervix. Concerned with survival and a sense of belonging to the human race, it is activated both at conception and when giving birth, bestowing a sense of 'earthing' and gravity to gestation and delivery. Awareness of this chakra is fundamental to all growth. Activated by standing and sitting postures.

Eating well

Pregnancy gives you the nose of a bloodhound and tastebuds of unusual sensitivity, but during the first trimester these will seem like a curse if you feel constantly nauseous. If you are vomiting or cannot eat much, you may worry that your baby is not receiving enough nourishment, but at this stage the baby is small enough to be getting sufficient nutrition, however sick you are. The nausea usually passes by the second trimester, the time you need to eat plenty of protein, and sensitive tastebuds will now make eating a pleasure.

Food cravings

You may find yourself desiring foods you normally don't eat, or an unusual mixture of foods. A craving to eat a non-food substance such as coal (called pica) is rare, but indicates that the body needs something in the substance craved – trace minerals, perhaps. If you long to eat refined, sugary food such as chocolate, you probably need the iron it contains, but you can satisfy this need just as well by eating grapes or raisins and other dried fruit. If you are a vegetarian and have a sudden desire for meat, try instead eating yeast extract on wholewheat bread, any soya bean preparation or food containing zinc, such as sweetcorn.

A well-balanced diet

Our diet today can be better and more balanced than ever before. If you are eating a well-balanced diet you won't need vitamin supplements, as vitamins are extracted much more easily and efficiently from food than from tablets. Since iron requirements are particularly high during pregnancy, iron tablets may be a useful standby, especially for vegetarians. If you do take iron tablets, make sure they are medically approved.

A developing foetus will take from the mother whatever it needs to develop, even if that will leave the mother short. Eating a healthy diet during pregnancy will ensure your baby receives all its bodybuilding requirements needed for a good start in life without draining you. It will also help your body deal with all the hormonal and physical changes of pregnancy. A well-balanced diet contains protein, fresh fruit and vegetables, a reasonable amount of fat and carbohydrates and plenty of water. Excessive cooking usually destroys vitamins, so eat vegetables raw or lightly steamed. An exception is in the case of potatoes, whose food value increases enormously with cooking. Carrots are more easily digested if lightly cooked or juiced.

Weight gain

The hormone progesterone slows down the metabolic rate, meaning that weight gain will be up to 50 per cent more than usual, especially during the second trimester. Fruit is a more healthy and efficient means of keeping the blood sugar levels high than foods containing fats, carbohydrates or refined sugar.

Live foods for life

Because you are nurturing young life, any 'live' foods will taste attractive. These include live yoghurt, alfalfa, bean sprouts, seeds and fresh vegetables.

Protein

Protein forms the essence of all living things, so naturally a pregnant mother needs plenty of it. Proteins consist of chains of amino acids and take different forms for different functions, such as holding the bones together, preventing disease or operating as enzymes. Well-known high-protein foods include meat, cheese and eggs, but these are also high in undesirable saturated fat. Few people realize just how much protein is found in such foods as wholewheat bread and sprouted alfalfa – more than in the best steak. Nuts, beans, pulses, seeds and any sprouted beans or seeds are healthy protein sources. Any food made from soya beans is high in protein, low in fat and rich in minerals.

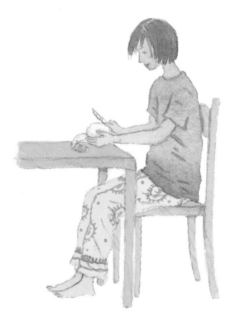

'As food is the body's first need, so it is proper nourishment which heals the body when it is sick. Those who recognize food as divine shall want for nothing.'

Taittyra Upanishad

Vitamins, fats and minerals

The following list describes the effects of essential vitamins, fats and minerals, and the best food sources.

VITAMINS
With few exceptions, the body cannot manufacture its own vitamins, and so must obtain them from food. A varied diet that includes a wide range of foods is likely to contain enough vitamins.

Vitamin A – the protector
• Strengthens the immune system and ensures healthy gums, skin and eyes.
• Found in butter, egg yolk, turnips, beetroot, yellow vegetables such as carrots and yams, yellow fruits such as mangoes, peaches, bananas, apricots, and green plants such as spinach, broccoli, Brussels sprouts and particularly parsley. Also in all fish oils, especially cod-liver oil.

Vitamin B complex
• All the vitamins of the B group are needed daily, to enable the body to perform its functions. A deficiency causes depression, nausea, constipation and heartburn. Yoghurt, though it does not contain vitamin B, helps assimilate it into the system. In turn, Vitamin B complex helps absorb calcium, found in yoghurt. Baking powder, coffee and sugar block assimilation.

Vitamin B1 – the tranquillizer
• Also known as thiamin, it counteracts depression by helping digestion, soothing the nervous system and promoting cell growth. Thiamin is destroyed by sodium, for which reason baking powder is not recommended for heartburn.
• Found in hazelnuts, peanuts, soya beans, whole grains, peas, bran, brown rice, cabbage and sprouts.

Vitamin B2 – the booster
• Also known as riboflavin, it is instrumental in breaking down carbohydrates, oxygenating cells, replacing and building up tissues.
• Found in milk, cheese, cottage cheese, cream, cereals, nuts, yeast, whole wheat, peas and beans. Also chicken.

Vitamin B5 – the energizer
• Boosts the immune system, increases energy and counteracts stress.
• Found in mushrooms, beans, brown rice and nuts.

Vitamin B6 – the sponge
• Aids protein absorption. Helps maintain hormonal balance, strengthens the nerves and reduces fluid retention.
• Found in avocados, green leafy vegetables such as cabbage, parsley and spinach. Also salmon and beef.

Vitamin B12 – the equalizer
• Aids the production of red blood cells. Especially important during pregnancy, since many more red blood cells are

What not to eat
A few foods are inadvisable during pregnancy. They include soft cheeses such as Brie, because of a possible link with listeria infection, and raw or lightly cooked eggs, such as in ice cream, because of the slight risk of salmonella poisoning. Salt intake should be minimal, since it can increase water retention and thus the blood pressure.

produced. It is said that vegetarians need to take this in a supplement form, and many prepared vegetarian foods contain added B12. The body is in fact able to produce its own vitamin B12, but the presence of meat in the colon kills off this natural source; therefore it is meat-eaters, or people who have recently become vegetarian, who should watch their intake.
• Found in eggs, dairy products and yeast extract. Also fish, oysters, pork, and beef.

Folic acid – the spine builder
• Needed for the absorption of iron and vital for the formation of the baby's central nervous system and spine in the first three months (a deficiency has been linked to spina bifida). As it also maintains blood volume, you will need about twice as much folic acid as usual throughout pregnancy. Because of its link with iron, a deficiency will also lead to anaemia. Excessive cooking can destroy folic acid, so it is best to eat the vegetables containing it either raw or lightly steamed. It may be taken in tablet form.
• Found in green foliage such as lettuce, spinach, kale and clover, as well as broccoli, milk, orange juice, potatoes, eggs and mushrooms.

Niacin – the fat reducer
• This vitamin improves the circulation of the blood, balances blood sugar and reduces cholesterol levels.
• Found in nuts, whole grains, eggs, soya beans, fish, meat and liver.

Vitamin C – the bloomer
• Also known as ascorbic acid, it keeps the gums healthy, clears the skin and nourishes the immune system. Needed daily, it also helps the body absorb iron. When eaten in the form of citrus fruits, it is easier for the body to assimilate if the whole fruit is eaten, rather than just the juice; this also balances the acid content and reduces heartburn and spots. Since this vitamin is water-soluble, wash lettuce leaves, for example, quickly under a running tap rather than by immersing in a bowl of water. Foods rich in iron aid absorption of vitamin C, whereas coffee and nicotine block absorption.
• Found in all citrus fruits such as oranges, lemons, limes and grapefruit, as well as strawberries, blackcurrants, watermelon, kiwi fruit, melons, tomatoes, green vegetables, carrots, radishes, peppers and potatoes.

Vitamin D – the sunshine
• Necessary for the absorption of calcium, which is needed for building the baby's bones, teeth and nervous system.
• Found in sunshine, butter, enriched margarine and milk. Also in fish oils and extracts and most animal fats.

Vitamin E – the skin builder
• Builds up and protects skin cells, helps supply oxygen to the tissues, and aids blood flow. The iron supplement ferrous sulphate destroys it.
• Found in beansprouts and all sprouting seeds, almonds, peanuts, butter, tomatoes, lettuce and eggs.

Vitamin K – the coagulant
• Necessary for blood clotting, and produced by the mother's body. As it does not pass easily through the placenta to the baby, however, it is usually given to newborn babies routinely, in order to counteract any haemorrhaging. It used to be injected, but as this has been found, in rare cases, to be dangerous, it is now more usually given orally.
• Found in green leafy vegetables, cauliflower, yoghurt, soya beans and eggs.

FATS
Fats provide a concentrated form of energy, and so are only needed in small amounts. There are two main types: saturates (mainly animal fats) and polyunsaturates.

Polyunsaturates – the friendly fats
• These break down other fats in the body and reduce cholesterol levels, helping to clean the heart as it undertakes the extra work of pregnancy.

• Found in fish oils, evening primrose oil, sesame seeds and all nuts except Brazil nuts.

MINERALS
Minerals are essential for the production of all the extra red blood cells, and the new tissues in the baby's body. Some, such as iron and calcium, are needed in larger than usual quantities during pregnancy; others, such as phosphorus and magnesium, are trace elements, and only needed in minute amounts.

Iron – the blood builder
• Sufficient iron is vital during pregnancy, since it is an essential ingredient of red blood cells, which supply you and your baby with oxygen. Your baby is also using up to a third of your intake in order to build up its own iron reserves. With an increased blood circulation you will notice if you are not getting enough. Iron deficiency causes symptoms of fatigue, dizziness and breathlessness, and can be confirmed by checking the insides of the lower eyelids. A pale pink indicates a deficiency, whereas a deep red colour is normal. It is usually better to eat iron-rich foods than take pills, which may cause or aggravate constipation. The body more easily absorbs iron if you eat it in conjunction with vitamin C, so, for example, eat your breakfast egg with a glass of orange juice. Caffeine blocks its absorption. Although chocolate contains iron, it also contains caffeine and sugar, which will reduce its efficiency. If iron is taken in the form of spinach, the spinach must be fresh, since iron will not keep if the spinach is cooked and then eaten the next day, and may even cause stomach upset.
• Found in green leafy vegetables, especially spinach, dried fruits such as apricots, raisins and prunes, nuts such as almonds, wholewheat bread, beetroot, mushrooms, eggs, peas, wheatgerm and cocoa. Also in sardines and all red meat, especially kidney and beef.

Calcium – the bone loader
• Essential for the formation of the baby's bones and teeth, so you will need to eat considerably more than usual. Also needed for normal muscle function and for strengthening and soothing the nervous system. It is a natural relaxant. To be assimilated, it must be eaten together with the vitamin B complex and poly-unsaturated fats. If you drink fat-free dairy products like skimmed milk, have it with fat of some sort in order that the body can absorb its calcium content efficiently.
• Found in dairy products, egg yolk, carrots, citrus fruits, prunes, seaweed, beansprouts, alfalfa sprouts, kale, broccoli, soya beans, sesame seeds, brewer's yeast, almonds, dried figs, carob and grains. Also in salmon and sardines.

Magnesium – the fat boss
• Helps the body cope with fats and carbohydrates, as well as aiding the absorption of protein. Stimulates heart function and circulation, and has a pacifying effect on the system.
• Found in green leafy vegetables, avocados, nuts, peas, all beans including soya beans, wheatgerm and all sprouted seeds and grains. Also in seafood.

Phosphorus – the smiler
• Needed for the absorption of calcium by the teeth and bones. Severe cramps in the calf muscles, usually at night, are a sign of an imbalance. Also helps the glands to function efficiently.
• Found in dairy products, onions, wholewheat bread, soya beans, peanuts and all whole grains. Also in tuna fish and white meat.

Potassium – the muscle worker
• Helps the heart and circulation, and keeps the muscles working properly. It also prompts many of the enzymes into action.
• Found in bananas, whole grains, vegetables, dried apricots, dates and prunes, elderberries and avocados.

Zinc – the brain builder
• Needed for brain formation and the healthy development of all tissues. It helps prevent nausea and plays a part in the healing process. Vegetarians are susceptible to zinc deficiency.
• Found in bananas, seeds, nuts, wheatgerm, sweetcorn, maize flour, tomatoes, carrots, bran and all whole grains and sprouted seeds. Also found in particularly high quantities in meat, fish and oysters.

Part two

The essential exercises

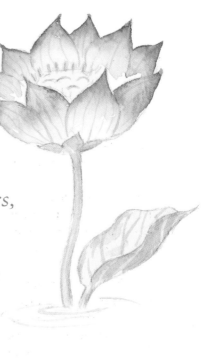

'Even as the lotus, loveliest of all the flowers,
has its roots deep down in the foulest slime
and opens her petals to the sun, so the
enlightened soul draws sustenance from the
darkness of human experience and, rising
above the turbulent waters, experiences the
transcendental joy of integration.'

Traditional Indian saying

CHAPTER THREE

Yoga for the first trimester

Even before there are any visible signs of pregnancy, enormous changes are taking place within you. These changes commonly cause fatigue and nausea during the first 12 weeks or so, until your body has had time to adjust to its new state. Rest as much as possible and allow your body to do its work. Resting can be done yogically, with breath awareness and the Corpse pose.

Although you may feel ready for yoga practice, don't do any active asanas during the first trimester because of the increased risk of miscarriage (see the caution, right). If you have not done yoga before, now is the time to cultivate breath awareness. You are breathing for your baby as well as yourself, and learning to breathe in a full and relaxed way will increase oxygen levels for both of you. Breathing well also enhances physical health, massaging the internal organs and stimulating circulation and digestion.

Breath is a vital ingredient of all yoga asanas, and instructions for breathing are given with every posture in this book. If you practise breath awareness daily during the first trimester, by the time you are ready to begin the asanas after 14 weeks, you will find that the breath will come naturally, in just the right place at just the right time, while you are doing the poses. Awareness of your breathing will also enable you to stay calm and centred during labour, allowing you to welcome the rhythm of the contractions instead of resisting it.

Savasana, or the Corpse – an integral part of every yoga session – is the pose for breathing exercises and for true relaxation. It will be of great benefit if practised daily now. Whatever your level of experience in yoga, this is also an excellent time to begin doing pelvic-floor exercises. These simple exercises, which may be done as visualizations, can help maintain the muscle tone of the pelvic floor and prevent problems associated with the extra weight of pregnancy and the stress of childbirth.

Caution: Don't do asanas (yoga poses) during the first trimester: extreme stretches and back bends, in particular, can dislodge the embryo, which may not yet be completely embedded in the uterine wall. In addition, your lowered blood pressure at this time may make you feel faint if you stand still for long. Raising your arms may cause tingling fingers, forward bends and deep breathing may make you dizzy and twists can cause nausea.

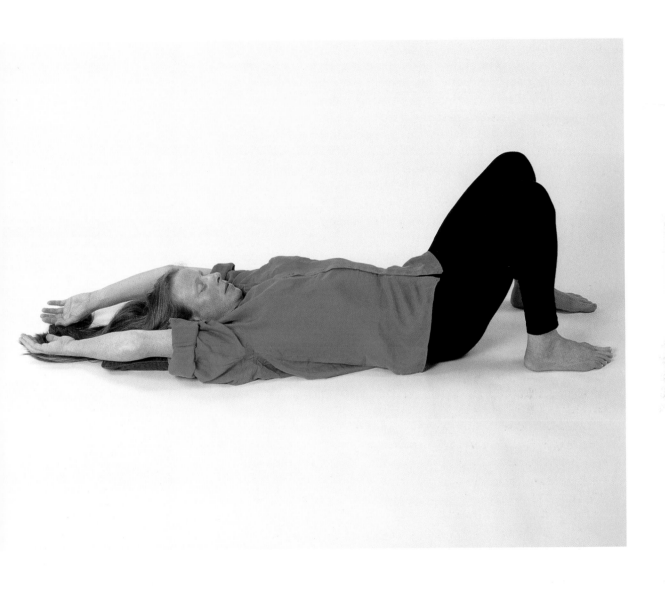

Breath awareness

Breath is the only vital function in the autonomic nervous system over which we can exercise direct, voluntary control. Breath is the link between the conscious and the unconscious, and awareness of the breath can be used to connect us to our subconscious, which guides our emotions and maintains, or returns us to, a state of harmony and tranquillity.

Before we can control the breath, it is essential first to become aware of it. By lying down in a safe environment and simply watching the breath – how it enters the lungs, how deeply it enters the lungs, how the diaphragm, ribcage and sternum move – we are taking the first steps towards eventual control. This process in itself relaxes the stomach muscles, sending back signals to the rest of the body to stimulate the calming response. The following simple exercises will help you become aware of your breathing. Do them whenever you have a few minutes of solitude to spare. Later, you will find it useful to do them before and after a yoga session. As well as helping you to relax into your body, they will help the breath come more easily while you are doing the asanas. Keep your breathing natural and light to begin with, but be aware of it at all times.

For detailed instructions on how to lie down, see the Corpse pose on page 43. To save you constantly referring to this book, have your partner or a friend read the instructions to you while you follow them, or tape them and play them back to yourself.

Begin by simply observing the breath, as described opposite, and practising relaxation. When you are accustomed to using your 'inner eyes' you can move on to breath control (Pranayama, pages 106–10).

Caution: During the first trimester you can lie flat as for the Corpse pose shown on page 43, but in the second and third trimesters, adapt to your growing uterus by always lying with your knees bent (as shown below) to prevent cutting off the blood return from your legs. If this position becomes uncomfortable, elevate your back by leaning against a beanbag (see right), making sure that your lower back, shoulders and head are well supported.

As you do the three-part breath, facing page, your hands may move apart as you inhale and move together as you exhale.

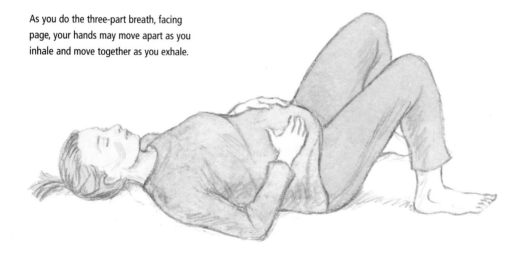

The three-part breath

Lie down comfortably (either flat on the floor or with support) with your knees bent. Roll back your shoulders and lengthen the back of your neck to prevent your chin sticking up. Place your hands on your abdomen so your middle fingers are touching just above the navel.

1 Feeling the diaphragm move

Observe your abdomen moving up into your hands as you inhale, and falling away as you exhale. Relax any tension out of your abdomen, and feel your baby moving gently down towards your spine as you exhale, and up to your hands as you inhale.

Become aware of your diaphragm, the wall of muscle separating the lungs from your internal organs. As your abdomen relaxes on the inhalation, the diaphragm expands, and you will feel the lungs opening up of their own accord, a little more with every breath.

Observe the breath for a few minutes.

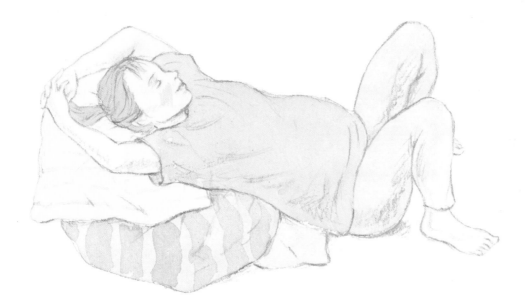

2 Feeling the ribcage move

Move your hands up and place the heels of your hands on the lower ribs so your middle fingers touch somewhere over the gap between the ribs.

Again, simply observe the breath for a few minutes. As you inhale, feel how the ribs separate. As you exhale, feel them closing together again. As you inhale again, be aware of how your whole ribcage rises and expands.

3 Feeling the sternum move

Place the palms of your hands lightly on your sternum – the upper part of your chest – with the middle fingers touching.

Breathe normally, and observe whether your hands rise and fall, slip apart, or stay still. (People vary in this.)

Spend a couple of minutes being aware of the fact that your lungs do reach up into the clavicular region.

When you are used to this exercise, you can rest your arms above your head, as shown above, and simply watch the flow of the breath.

Arm extensions

Arm extensions help to open up the lungs completely, including the upper, clavicular region. They also relieve tired shoulders, and so you will find them especially useful after the birth, as a counterpoise to breast-feeding and bending over the baby.

Lying with your back flat on the floor and your knees bent, bring your arms down by your sides, palms facing upwards.

Squeeze your shoulder blades together so you open up the 'eyes' of the shoulders. Lie still, breathe normally, and turn your palms down.

On an inhalation, raise one arm in the air and bring it back through a semicircle to rest on the floor behind you. If your shoulders or elbows are stiff and do not lie comfortably flat, support them with a cushion. Lie still and relax the arm, breathing normally for a couple of breaths. Feel the armpit opening and softening.

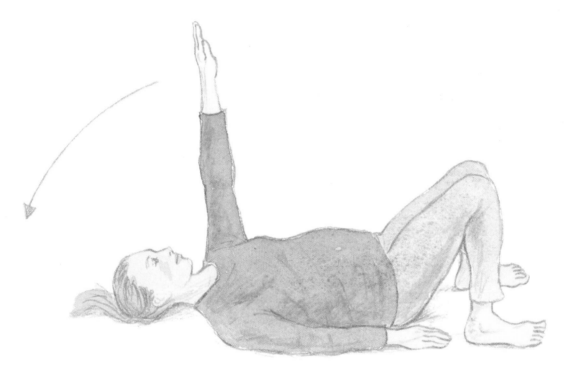

Inhale, stretching the arm along the floor away from you, and on the exhalation, return your arm through the semicircle to rest on the floor beside you again.

Repeat on the other side and then twice more on each side.

Try doing the same exercise using both arms together.

The Corpse pose

This is the best pose in which to relax, breathe and meditate. If done regularly and sincerely, it can remove the worries of the world from your shoulders. It purifies the circulation and leaves you feeling refreshed, light and buoyant, however big you are. Cleansed of negative thoughts, you will feel more active, alert and happy. Even if you have no time for any other yoga, it is worth making time for the Corpse.

The Corpse, or Savasana, is the traditional way to start and finish a yoga session. Beginning with it is optional, but finishing with it is vital, in order to calm the mind and body and to 'seal' the differences that yoga has made. Make sure you are warmly covered if the room is cool, because the Corpse does not involve any active stretching and the body temperature will drop. If possible, make sure that you are alone, and will not be disturbed. Dim or turn off bright lights, and prepare to relax.

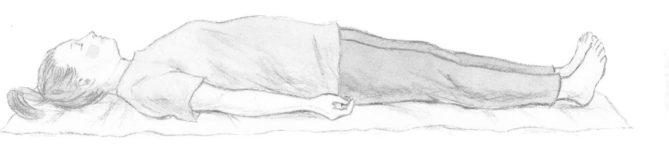

Lying down for the Corpse

You can lie flat in the first trimester, but you will need to adjust this position as your pregnancy advances, either bending your knees or supporting your back, or both.

Without straining your back, gently lie down on your back on the floor, making sure that your head, neck and spine are all in a straight line.

Stretch your legs out flat on the floor, with the ankles apart, and extend the heels so the toes are pointing to the ceiling. Relax the feet, so they fall outward slightly.

Relaxation in the Corpse

Clenching and relaxing progressive sets of muscles throughout the body help you focus on them and, conversely, to let go – in every sense of the word. Clench on the exhalation each time, and hold it for two or three seconds, as hard as you can. Inhale, breathe normally for a breath, and move on to the next part of the body. Do not hold your breath at any stage.

Start with your toes: clench them hard as you exhale, and let go. Lift the arches of your feet, turn the toes up, and let go. Tense your calves, and let go. Draw your kneecaps back, very hard – and let go. Tense your thigh muscles, front and back – and let go.

Clench your buttocks, and release. Draw the whole network of your pelvic floor upwards – and let go. Contact and contract all the muscles holding your uterus up, attaching it to your spine. Clench, and let go.

Hunch your shoulders high up to your ears, and let go. Clench your upper arms, very hard, and let go. Clench your lower arms, and let go.

Make fists of your hands, holding your thumbs inside – clench, and release. Tighten all the muscles in your neck, clench your teeth together, and let go. Open your jaw as wide as it will go, straining the hinges, and let go. Wrinkle your nose like a rabbit, and let go. Screw up your eyes as if the lids were tissue paper, and let go. Raise your eyebrows, corrugate your forehead and feel your scalp moving – and let go.

Breathe normally for a couple of minutes, savouring the levity. Now inhale, and at the same time, clench the whole of your legs from your toes to your buttocks.

Without a pause, exhale and simultaneously release your legs and clench your pelvic floor. Do not clench your abdomen.

Inhale, and clench your neck, shoulders, arms, hands and head.

Exhale, and release your whole body.

Relax completely for a few minutes before coming up slowly, as described on page 45.

If lying flat in the Corpse pose is uncomfortable, support your head and back on cushions or a beanbag, as shown.

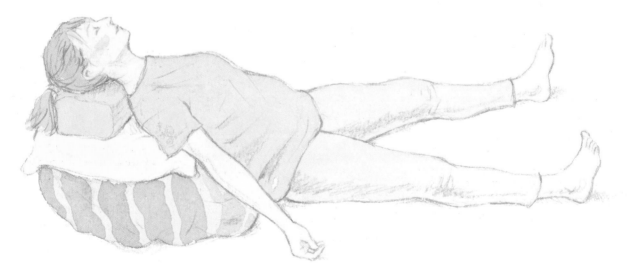

Body of light

Rather than trying to remember this relaxation exercise, have your partner or a friend read the instructions to you, or read them into a tape-recorder and play them back to yourself. You may also like to play soothing background music. Leave appropriate spaces between each visualization – the symbol § represents approximately one minute.

Lie down comfortably and focus on the natural rise and fall of the breath. §

Feel your belly soft, warm, giving, open and relaxed, and visualize your baby rising and falling with the breaths. §§

Take three deep breaths, the out-breath being longer than the in-breath. §§

Now be aware that when we breathe, we take in not only air but also prana. Prana is life energy, and we can visualize it as a dancing white light. Watch it softly entering your nostrils, flowing down your air passages to the thousands of tiny air-sacs in your lungs; feel the light percolating through your lungs, gathering at your heart and moving outwards in waves throughout your body. §

In a wave of light it flows down, through your abdomen, around your baby, through your hips, your thighs, your knees, your shins, your calves, your ankles, right down to the soles of your feet. Feel the soles of your feet, very wide and open, radiant with light, and feel the energy flowing to the tips of your toes. Feel the spaces between your toes, feel your toenails growing. §

Bring your attention back to your breath. Again, focus on the breath, visualize the white dancing light flowing softly down into your lungs, gathering at your heart and flooding out now through your shoulders, down through your upper arms, your elbows and your wrists. Feel the palms of your hands, very open and light, capable and radiant. Feel the light flowing through all the joints of your fingers, feel the spaces between your fingers and feel the light dancing on your fingertips. §

Again, bring your focus back to your breath, and watch the wave of light now streaming up through your neck, your throat and into your jaw. Feel it moving around your gums, in your teeth, through your tongue and out to your ears. Feel your ears, alert and yet relaxed, and watch the wave of light moving through your sinuses to your nostrils and up to your eyes. Feel your eyes very soft and light, as if resting in a sea of liquid light, and feel the skin around your eyes soft and gentle, every pore open and yielding. Feel the light moving up now to your forehead, opening up your third eye. Be aware of the light moving softly through your scalp, nourishing the root of every hair on your head, and take your mind deep into your mind. Feel the prana flushing through your brain, washing through every neuron and thought process. §

Again, bring your focus back to your breath, and watch it expanding gently throughout your being. You feel very light, light as a balloon. §§

Visualize a wave of white dancing light now moving down to your baby, surrounding her in a protective aura of energy and love. Feel your baby secure in her own world. §

Now feel the space between you and your baby. Visualize the light again, encircling your baby, keeping both of you safe, simultaneously connected and separate. §

Now bring your focus back to your breath. As you breathe in, draw in the energy and light, and breathe out with a sensation of letting go of any shadows. You are bathed in vitality, peace and well-being. Breathe in with a sense of freedom, and breathe out with a sense of release. §§§

Coming up

Come up slowly, spending several minutes over it. Begin by wiggling your fingers and toes; then stretch your arms over your head, and stretch in whatever way feels comfortable. Roll over on to your side, and rest your head on your hand. Open your eyes when you feel ready, and come up in your own time. Do not leap right back into normal life – reintegrate slowly, if you can. This will be kinder to your nervous system and the benefits of the relaxation will be deeper and longer lasting.

The pelvic floor

The pelvic floor, as its name suggests, is the layer of muscles that lines the base of the pelvis. These muscles form a 'hammock' extending from the base of the spine to the base of the pubic bone. There are three outlets in the pelvic floor: the anus, the vagina and the urethra, which are held closed by rings of muscle, or sphincters. The pelvic floor supports the weight of all the body's organs, and during pregnancy the effects of hormonal changes combined with the pressure of the enlarging uterus may slow the pelvic circulation, leading to congestion and discomfort.

The extra weight of pregnancy and the stress of childbirth may weaken the pelvic-floor muscles, particularly the sphincter of the urethra, causing involuntary leakage of urine under pressure. During childbirth, the main muscles of the pelvic floor are pushed aside by the widening of the vagina as the baby emerges. The muscles will go back to their original position but may be slackened by the process, especially in a second or subsequent delivery. After the birth, the vaginal walls may also lose some of their elasticity.

Pelvic-floor exercises

Fortunately, simple exercises can, if performed daily throughout pregnancy, maintain the tone of the pelvic-floor muscles and may even make them better than before. Pelvic-floor exercises will help prevent problems associated with the stretching of these muscles during childbirth. The exercises will not only prevent urine leakage (stress incontinence) and allow you to continue to have a satisfying sex life, but will also, by stimulating the blood supply, reduce the likelihood of a tear, speed up the healing process after the birth and reduce the risk of complications such as a prolapsed uterus or haemorrhoids.

Pelvic-floor exercises are most effective if done regularly while you are pregnant, and are especially helpful in the last month when the muscles are most stressed. They should also be done after the birth, gently at first if you have had stitches and are uncomfortable, and become a lifelong habit. Because they are so simple it is easy to forget to do them, but experience will show you that they work. No one can see what you are doing, so you can do them at any time, anywhere. If you make a habit of doing them at the same time as, for example, watching television or drinking tea, the other activity can act as a trigger. The number of times a day you do them depends on your muscle tone. Start by doing as many as you can comfortably, and gradually build on that number until you are doing up to a hundred daily.

Pelvic-floor visualizations

These strengthening exercises help you focus on the correct muscles of the pelvic floor, and familiarize you with the sensation of contracting and releasing them.

The pelvic lift

This one uses the whole pelvic floor

Imagine you have a friend who lives on the sixth floor. The building has no lift so you must use the stairs, resting on each floor. There are two flights of stairs between each floor.

Sit, stand or squat comfortably. Inhale evenly, and visualize yourself ascending the first flight of stairs. As you do so, contract the muscles of your pelvic floor. When you are halfway through your inhalation, imagine you have turned to ascend the second flight.

As you go up the second half, contract your muscles even harder, as hard as you possibly can.

Exhale evenly, visualizing yourself resting on the first landing as you relax your pelvic floor.

Inhale, and visualize yourself ascending to the next floor.

Continue until you reach the top.

Vaginal squeezes

By concentrating on your vagina, you focus on its two sets of muscles: the sphincter, which keeps it closed, and the folded muscle of the vaginal walls. In this exercise you contract the muscles while exhaling, not when inhaling, which means that you can incorporate it into any position that involves turning the tailbone under (see page 51). You can also test the exercise's effectiveness during sexual intercourse.

Inhale deeply and, on the exhalation, slowly contract the muscles of the vaginal passage only, drawing them in and up. Inhale, and relax.

Repeat ten times, increasing the number of repetitions as you become proficient.

Anal squeezes

Imagine you are trying to hold in wind in a potentially embarrassing situation, and draw together the muscles of the anal sphincter with increasing strength. Inhale evenly, contracting the anus as you do so. Let the vagina and urethra remain relaxed.

Exhale evenly, relaxing the anal sphincter and surrounding muscles.

Repeat several times.

Urethral squeezes

To discover the correct muscles to use, start by doing the exercise while urinating.

As you begin to urinate, count to two and then contract your muscles until you stop the flow. When it has stopped, let it go again and count to two.

Repeat the contractions until your bladder is empty. If at first you are unable to stop the flow of urine, do not give up; you will find that with practice your muscle control will improve tremendously.

As you exhale, focus on drawing up the muscles around the urethra. Visualize yourself lifting up the bladder as you do so.

Caution: Because of the slightly increased risk of urinary infection, do not do this exercise more than once a day while urinating. You can try it 'dry' any time.

CHAPTER FOUR

Yoga for the second trimester

The second trimester of pregnancy lasts from about the 14th until the 28th week. The nausea and fatigue of the early weeks usually diminish and disappear, and you begin to acquire an aura of vitality. This is the time to enjoy daily yoga exercise, choosing from the sequences described in this chapter.

Your ligaments and muscles are more supple than usual, and you should now be able to do all the yoga asanas, or postures, recommended for pregnancy. You will need to adapt your practice, however, as the uterus grows. Leaning forward will become progressively more difficult, so widen your stance for standing forward bends, and increase the distance between the diaphragm and pelvis by placing your hands on a chair or similar support rather than reaching right down as you usually would. This will give space to the growing baby. In sitting forward bends, extend the lower vertebrae so that you come forward but not down. In later months use a cushion, beanbag or chair on which to rest your head, hands and shoulders.

After the fourth month, pressure from the expanding uterus can cut off the blood return to the torso from the legs via the inferior vena cava (one of two large veins into which all the venous blood drains). For this reason it is not a good idea either to stand still in one position for any length of time, or to lie flat on your back with your legs stretched out. When resting or sleeping, facilitate blood flow either by lying on your side, supporting your upper knee with cushions, or, if you prefer to be supine, by elevating the back and head or bending the knees up.

When you stand, the increasing weight of the uterus will pull the stomach and upper back forward, putting a strain on the lower back and making backache more likely. Many yoga positions help to counteract this problem, including pelvic tilts against a wall or door, the Cat and its variations, squats, modified forward bends and gentle twists.

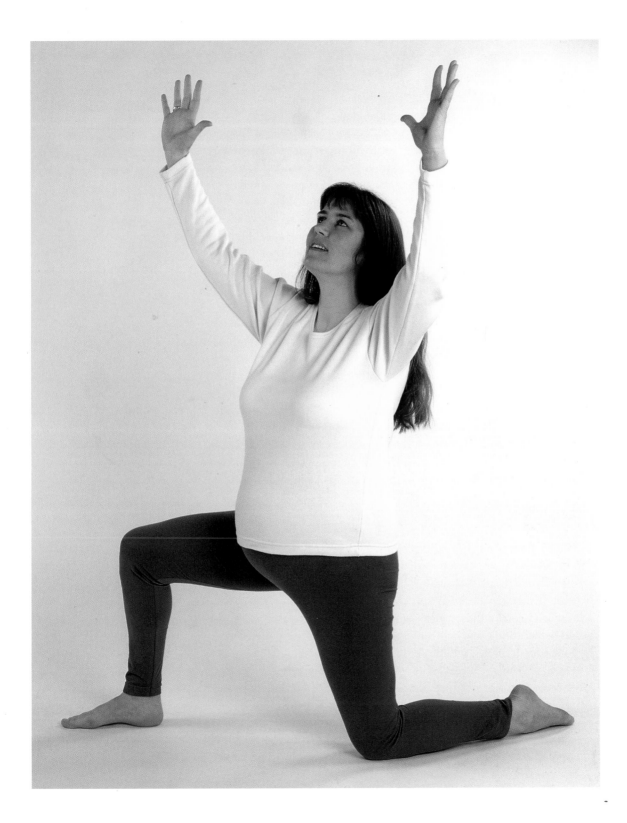

Your daily programme

The postures described on the following pages have been arranged in sequences, mostly according to the best time of day to do them, but they may be done at other times if you prefer. Factors such as how busy you are and, most importantly, how you feel, will determine when you do the sequences. Adapt them according to your circumstances. For example, if it is morning but you feel tired, do an evening programme. If you have limited time, omit the postures marked as optional.

Once you are familiar with the positions, or if you are experienced in yoga, you can make up your own sequences, making sure that you vary the asanas so that the whole body is stretched and toned. In the morning, or whenever you are feeling energetic, begin with lunges and standing poses. These get you moving, ready for the day ahead. Do not do too many or hold any position for longer than 30 seconds unless otherwise stated. Intersperse lively poses with the Cat and then move on to more calming positions, such as sitting forward bends. Follow forward bends with a gentle twist. Shoulder openers and neck looseners can be done at any point, in either a standing or sitting position.

Always finish off with a breathing exercise and relaxation. The breathing exercises suggested in the sequences are described fully in chapter 3 and in the section on more advanced breath control (Pranayama) on page 106. If you do not have much time, do only one asana of each type, but always include relaxation, which is important for instilling the benefit of the postures into your being.

Breathing

All asanas 'float' on the breath, and instructions for breathing are given with each one. If you have been practising breath awareness daily during the first trimester, you will probably find that the breath comes naturally as you do the poses. If you are new to yoga, however, it is better to breathe normally than try to remember exactly how and when you should be breathing with the movements. You may find yourself holding your breath, which will do more harm than good.

Breath is an integral part of all yoga practice, not just during the active poses but as a separate exercise at the end of each session. Breath awareness re-establishes the natural rhythm of the breath, while Pranayama is active breath control, and forms a bridge between the external and internal approaches to yoga. With practice the breath will slow and deepen, although deep breathing is not the aim. The aim is to expand the lungs gently and fully, and to focus especially on lengthening the out-breath.

Caution: Inverted poses are unsafe because the placenta is usually attached to the top of the uterus, and inversion will cause the baby's weight to press on the umbilical cord and restrict its oxygen supply. Shoulder stands are also unsuitable during pregnancy even if you are used to doing them, since they can raise the blood pressure. A full list of poses contra-indicated during pregnancy is given on page 24.

Touching base – an easy morning stretch

This sequence contains the basic moves upon which the rest of your practice depends. The standing postures, which are both invigorating and grounding, literally get you on your feet. They are good to do in the morning, as they dispel inertia and energize you for the coming day.

1 Pelvic tilt – 'turning the tailbone under'

Tilting the pelvis so that the tailbone (coccyx) 'turns under' unravels points of tension in the spine, counteracting the forward pull of the uterus in the later months.

Bend your knees and place your hands, palms down, on your lower back. As you exhale, stroke your hands down over your pelvis, allowing it to tilt so that your tailbone lengthens down.

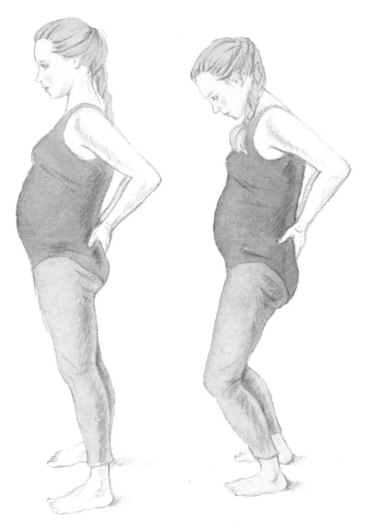

THE FEET

Well-placed feet make a solid foundation for all standing poses. For most of the simple standing positions, place the feet hip-width apart with the outsides parallel to one another and facing forwards.

Spread out all the toes, even the little ones. If you find moving the little toes difficult, practise in bare feet by interlocking your fingers with your toes and easing them backwards and forwards.

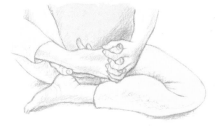

Distribute your weight evenly over the soles of your feet. Rock gently from side to side, backwards and forwards, and gently come to a standstill. Lift the arches and be aware of where and how your feet are coming into contact with the floor. Feel the feet widening downwards, and the rest of your body rising firm and light from its support.

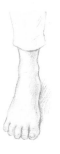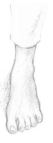

2 Hip circles

When you are pregnant, your centre of gravity moves down into the pelvic region, domain of the Svadhisthana chakra – which, translated, means 'one's own abode'. The pelvis is the cradle in which we were all once rocked, so as you do this exercise, gently create a region of awareness there, while loosening your hips.

Stand with your feet about hip-width apart. Place your hands on your hips and, keeping the knees loose, rotate your hips clockwise five or six times. Repeat in an anti-clockwise direction.

3 Simple lunge

This simple movement releases the lower back, opens the shoulders and stretches the heels in preparation for squatting.

Stand facing a wall, toes 8-12 inches away from it. Step one foot back, bend the leading knee and keep the back leg straight, with both heels on the floor. Toes and hips face forwards.

Lean your forearms and head against the wall. As you exhale, feel the calf and heel of the back leg lengthening. Hold for a minute, breathing easily. Repeat on the other side.

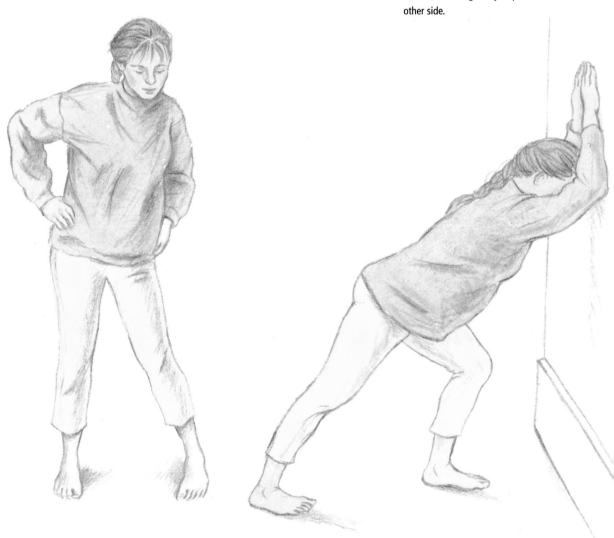

4 The Mountain

The Mountain (Tadasana) may seem static, but it is internally active. As well as instilling good posture, it is both serene and dynamic, and acts as a foundation for all the other standing postures.

Caution: Don't do the Mountain pose for more than a minute at a time.

Stand with your feet hip-width apart, outsides of the feet parallel, knees straight and the pelvis tilted. As you exhale, draw your kneecaps back, lengthen the hamstrings and thighs, and turn the tailbone under.

As you inhale, lift your spine and sternum, but don't puff out the chest, which may cause the lumbar spine to arch. Feel the chest expanding and the sternum opening.

Flatten your shoulder blades and, as you exhale, drop the shoulders, extend your arms and fingers downwards, and feel the distance between your shoulders and chin lengthening. Be aware of your head resting gently on top of your spine. Look straight ahead and internalize your attention, focusing on your centre of gravity.

Identify with your spine and draw all your energies inward to this central axis, the core of the mountain.

Be straight but not rigid: a dropped chin and straight spine invite clarity and humility. Soften your core and breathe the softness through you. You are a mountain, serene, firmly rooted, self-confident and self-contained.

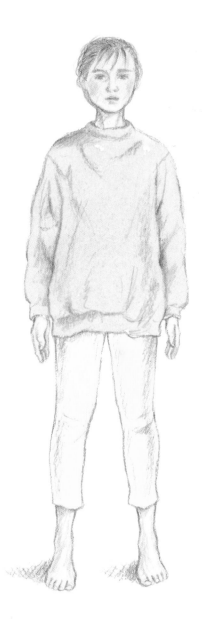

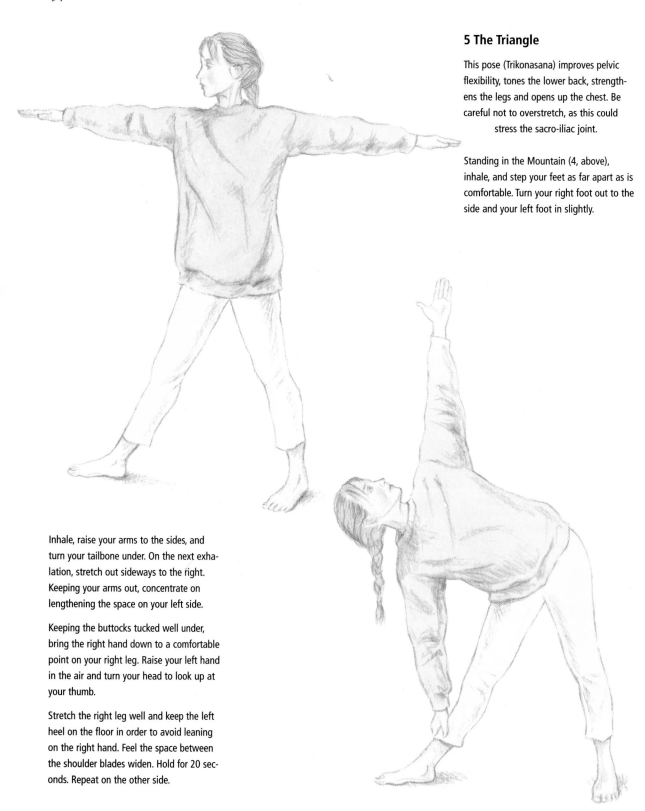

5 The Triangle

This pose (Trikonasana) improves pelvic flexibility, tones the lower back, strengthens the legs and opens up the chest. Be careful not to overstretch, as this could stress the sacro-iliac joint.

Standing in the Mountain (4, above), inhale, and step your feet as far apart as is comfortable. Turn your right foot out to the side and your left foot in slightly.

Inhale, raise your arms to the sides, and turn your tailbone under. On the next exhalation, stretch out sideways to the right. Keeping your arms out, concentrate on lengthening the space on your left side.

Keeping the buttocks tucked well under, bring the right hand down to a comfortable point on your right leg. Raise your left hand in the air and turn your head to look up at your thumb.

Stretch the right leg well and keep the left heel on the floor in order to avoid leaning on the right hand. Feel the space between the shoulder blades widen. Hold for 20 seconds. Repeat on the other side.

6 Standing forward bend

The free forward extension of this pose (Uttanasana) encourages blood flow to the legs and pelvis, and helps relieve the spine of the weight of the uterus. It also expands the abdomen and lungs, creating more space and oxygen for you and the baby.

Caution: Do not take your head below your waist if you have high blood pressure.

Stand in the Mountain (4, above) facing a hip-height support such as a window-ledge or the back of a chair. Inhale, raise your hands up above your head and, on the exhalation, put your hands on your hips. On the next exhalation, bend your torso forward, leading with the sternum and releasing from the base of the spine.

Stretch your arms in front of you so your hands rest lightly, shoulder-width apart, on the support. Keep the stomach long and soft, the toes well spread and the heels on the ground.

Your legs should be vertical. Keep extending from the base of the spine. With your head between your arms, look down.

Maintain the position for several breaths, or as long as is comfortable.

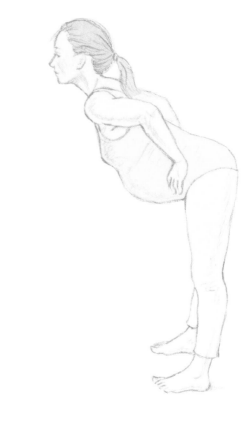

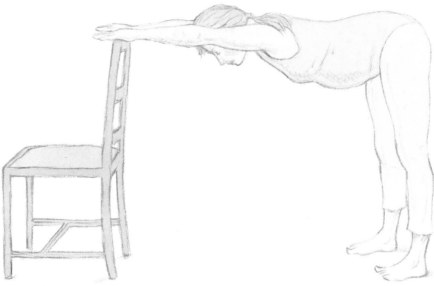

7 The Cat

The Cat pose relieves the pressure of the uterus on the lower back and the pelvic floor, allowing blood to circulate without stricture.

Caution: Do not allow the spine to sag in this position.

Go down on all fours. Hands should be shoulder-width apart, knees and ankles hip-width apart.

With your middle fingers parallel, spread your hands and press down evenly. Keep your head level with your spine, your spine parallel with the floor, and look down.

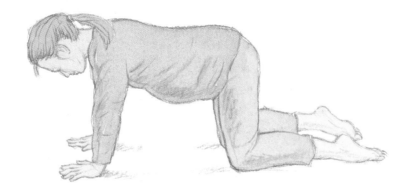

As you exhale, drop your head, tuck your tailbone under and hump your back like an angry cat.

As you inhale, return to the straight position.

As you exhale, again hump the back. Turn your pelvis under, feel your baby move up to your spine and feel the vertebrae separating.

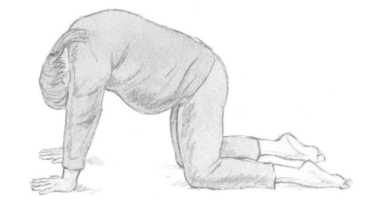

8 Squat

This pose creates more room for the baby, opens up the pelvis and stretches the lower back. If your feet will not go flat, use blocks or a rolled blanket under your heels. For extra support, sit on blocks, cushions or a low stool or lean against a wall.

Caution: Don't do this pose if you are more than 32 weeks pregnant and your baby is in the breech position.

Exhale, and drop into a squat, turning the toes out slightly.

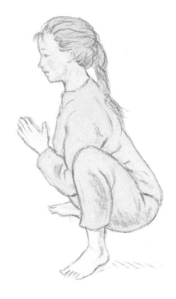

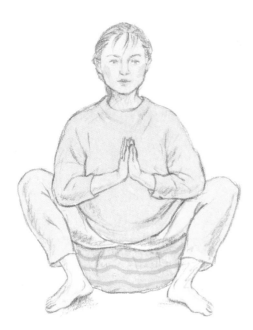

Place your hands together in the prayer position, and gently push your knees sideways with your elbows as you inhale, expanding your chest and lifting your lower ribs up and away from the baby. As you exhale, lengthen your tailbone downwards.

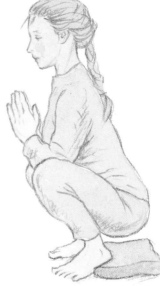

Lift the arches of your feet, spread the toes and press the outsides of the feet down. Direct your breathing towards the baby, visualizing the breath entering at your navel, bathing him or her with light energy.

Hold this for as long as is comfortable.

9 Seated angle pose

This wonderful pose, called Upavista Konasana, improves pelvic circulation and opens up the lower back. It will also relieve an aching symphysis pubis, the joint at the front of the pelvis, during later pregnancy.

Sit on the floor with your legs as far apart as they will go without straining, at the same angle as each another. Stretch into your heels and press the backs of the legs to the floor.

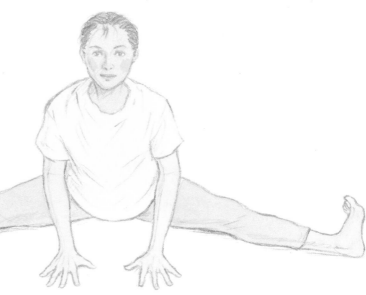

Inhale and lift up your arms, looking up. Feel the lift from the base of your spine reaching lightly right up to your fingertips.

On the exhalation, float your arms down in front of you. releasing your spine.

Maintain this pose, with adequate breathing, for as long as is comfortable. As the stretching relaxes the legs you will be able to open them more – but take care not to strain them.

10 Child's pose

This is extremely relaxing, simple, and can be done at any time. It stretches the back, tones the leg muscles and opens the shoulders. Put a block or cushion under your buttocks if necessary.

Kneel on the floor, knees apart and toes together. Sit on or between your feet.

Slide your hands forward along the floor on an exhalation, without lifting your buttocks.

Stretch forward on the in-breaths, opening up the shoulders. As you exhale, move the tailbone down towards the floor.

Hold for a minute or for as long as you feel comfortable.

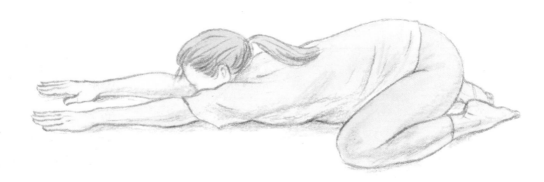

11 The Thunderbolt

This position is very compact, grounding and powerful – like a thunderbolt. Practised daily, the pose combats flat or tired feet.

Caution: This asana, done for short periods, may help prevent varicose veins, but if you already have them, avoid it.

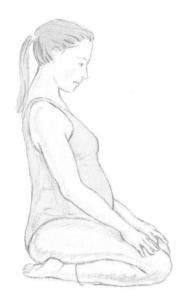

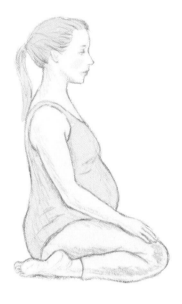

Kneel with your thighs together and sit back on your heels with your toes pointing straight back. Rest your hands on your thighs and breathe evenly. Drop your chin slightly.

If you are comfortable, slide your feet out from under you and sit between them. Press the tops of your feet to the ground and point the toes straight back. Rest your hands on your thighs and look straight ahead.

Visualize your tailbone as a taproot, growing down into the earth. Lift from the base of your spine and open your sternum on the inhalation, dropping the shoulders on the exhalation.

Try to keep your thighs together and maintain for a couple of minutes, breathing evenly.

If your legs tingle or feel uncomfortable, sit on a block, bolster, cushion or special 'Zen' stool. Omit the pose if you have weak knees. If your ankles are stiff, kneel with both legs on a pillow but your feet touching the floor.

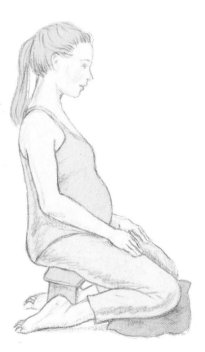

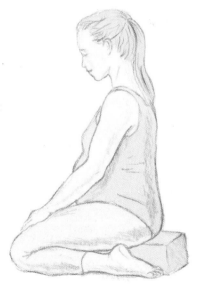

12 The Tailor's pose

So called because it is the pose of Indian tailors, this position, Baddha Konasana, tones the pelvic floor, increases the blood supply to the whole pelvic area including the bladder, and eases tension in the leg joints. Do this pose for as long as is comfortable.

Sit on the floor, bend the knees and bring the soles of the feet together. Hold the feet and draw the heels towards you.

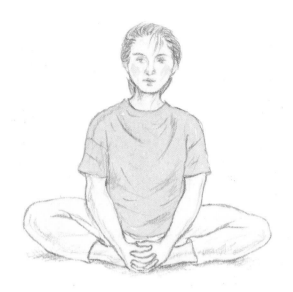

Gently place your hands on your knees and allow the knees to drop toward the floor.

Breathe your tailbone down into the floor. Open the abdomen, drop the shoulders and stretch the spine upwards.

If necessary, support the knees with rolled blankets or cushions. (To extend the pose, place your hands on the floor in front of you and, keeping the elbows bent, reach forward from the base of your spine on the out-breath for four or five breaths.)

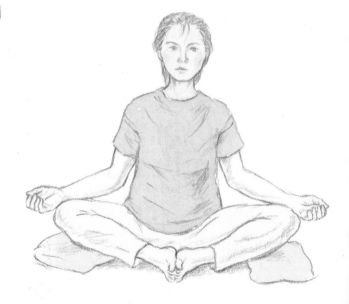

13 Simple sitting twist

Twists help relieve lower backache, open up the shoulders, help digestion, dispel constipation and enhance vitality.

From the Thunderbolt position (11, above), place your left hand on your right knee.

Place your right hand on the floor close to your right buttock. If you find yourself leaning, put your hand on a block or book.

Keeping your spine upright, inhale, and lift up. As you exhale, look over your right shoulder. As you inhale, untwist your head slightly and lift up as your lungs fill with air. Feel the left shoulder lengthening away from your chin.

Maintain the pose for a minute at most, and then repeat on the other side.

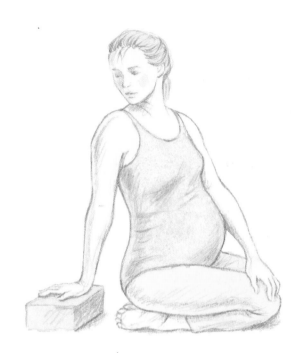

14 Neck crescents

This neck-loosening pose will relieve tension and ease headaches and shoulder-aches as well as neck-ache. As you do it, relax your shoulders and face as well as your neck, and try to empty your head too.

Sit upright in any comfortable position. Inhale, and on the exhalation, turn your head to the right, keeping the neck upright and the spine vertical. Inhale, and on the next exhalation describe a downward arc with your chin, dipping over the sternum.

Bring the chin up over the left shoulder, so that your skull is again vertically over the spine. Repeat three times each way.

Finish the sequence with relaxation in the Corpse pose (page 44).

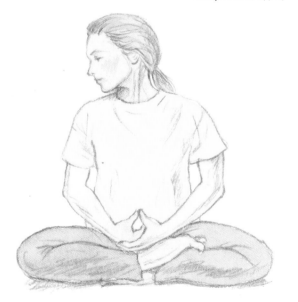

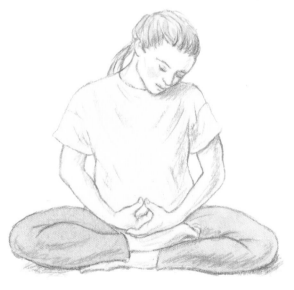

Dusting off the day – an easy evening stretch

This sequence of mainly sitting postures is suitable for the evening, or whenever you feel tired. It shakes off the dust of the day with calming positions, which you can hold for longer than standing asanas. There are fewer poses in the sequence than in some others, giving you more time to finish with soothing breath and relaxation in the Corpse.

1 Supine against a wall

Lying with your feet up against a wall eases congestion of the leg veins and relieves tired feet. Even when you feel too tired to do any exercise, this will refresh you. After about the fifth month, move your buttocks away from the wall or elevate them using a support, or both.

Caution: After 34 weeks or if you are uncomfortable, omit this exercise.

Legs straight up

Sit beside a wall. Lie down and, using your arms and not your stomach muscles, swivel round so your back is at right angles to the wall and your legs straight up.

Bring your arms above your head and rest them on the floor. Relax completely, and remain in this position as long as you like.

Soles of the feet together

Bring the soles of your feet together and, as you exhale, gently press your knees against the wall. Relax, and hold for as long as you like. To come up, roll on to your side, rest there for a moment, and come up on your hands and knees.

Legs apart

Slide your legs apart as far as they will go. Flex your ankles so that the backs of your knees are stretched. Hold for as long as is comfortable.

2 The Cat

See page 56.

3 Swaying Cat

In the Cat position, keep your arms straight and sway your hips from side to side, describing a crescent shape without dipping.

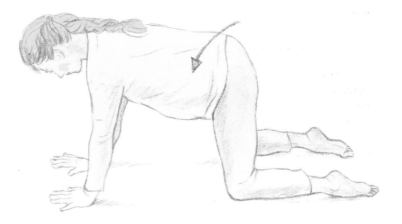

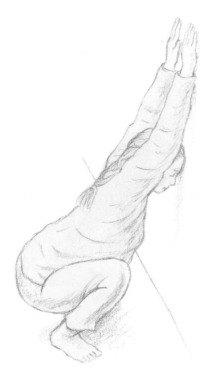

4 Squatting facing a wall

This opens the shoulders as well as the hips. Leaning into a wall provides more stability for squatting, making it easier to lengthen the lower back. If you can't rest down on your heels, support them with a rolled blanket or block.

Stand 12 inches away from the wall with your feet hip-width apart and tailbone under. Inhale, and on the exhalation, drop into a squat, turning the toes out slightly.

Raise your arms and place your forehead, hands and forearms flat on the wall.

As you inhale, draw your chest towards the wall and gently straighten your elbows. As you exhale, lower your tailbone to the floor.

Hold for a minute or two, or as long as is comfortable.

5 Leg circles

This is an effortless way of opening up the hips and so promoting blood flow to the whole pelvic region.

Caution: Though you may find it easier than usual to do so, don't bring the bent leg back too far – overstretching may damage the sacro-iliac joint. To overcome this problem, lean against a wall.

Lie on your right side so that your torso, thighs and lower legs form a `Z' shape. Support your head with your right hand, or use cushions if you prefer, especially in the later months.

Bend your left leg and describe circles in the air with your knee – clockwise and anti-clockwise – for about 30 seconds.

Repeat on the other side.

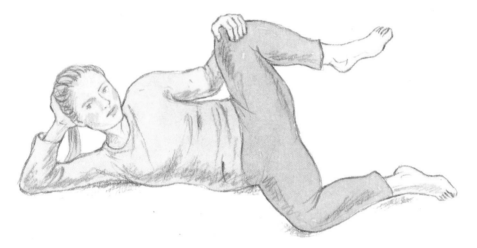

6 Seated forward bend

Forward bends are relaxing and calming. They help relieve insomnia, tone the kidneys and abdominal organs, and encourage pelvic circulation. Increase the stretch by using a belt looped round your foot.

Sit with your legs in front of you. Bring the right leg up, so the knee is bent to the side and the sole of the foot rests against the left thigh. Make sure the sacrum area is flat; if the right side moves back, bring the right foot further toward the knee.

Loop a belt around your left foot and, on the exhalation, extend from the base of your spine, as for a standing forward bend (see page 55). Maintain for two minutes or for as long as is comfortable. Repeat on the other side.

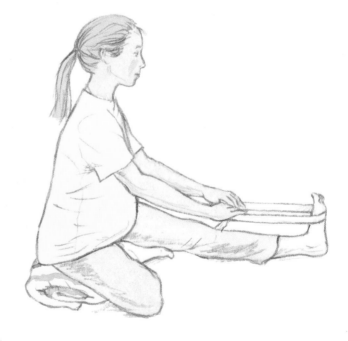

7 Sitting twist on a chair

Like the simple twist on page 61, this pose rotates the spine and helps relieve backache. It also improves digestion.

Sit sideways on an armless chair with its back to your right and your feet parallel. If your feet do not go flat on the floor, place blocks or books under them.

Inhale, and, lifting up from the base of your spine, place your hands either side of the chair-back.

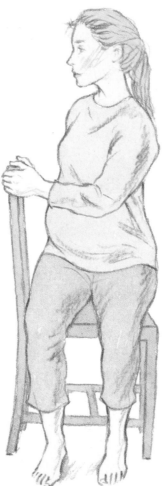

Drop your shoulders and feel the energy run right down through them rather than being blocked by a hunch.

Exhale, and turn your head to look over your right shoulder. Twist and stretch your lower back so it remains upright.

As you inhale, release the twist slightly and focus on lengthening the spine upwards. Exhale, and turn again and look over your right shoulder, visualizing the energy spiralling up your spine.

Hold for three breaths and repeat on the other side.

8 Seated Mountain pose

The chest expansion of this pose allows more air to circulate through the lungs, and the lift gives extra space to your baby. It also helps reduce swelling in the ankles and wrists.

Choose any comfortable sitting position. It may help to do the pose against a wall.

Interlock the fingers and stretch your arms out straight in front of you, turning the palms away from you.

Inhale, and stretch them up above your head. Keep the sternum open and your shoulder blades moving into your back.

Extend the palms to the ceiling. Open up the armpits and keep a straight spine, lifting up from the floor to your palms.

Hold it for no longer than 30 seconds.

Change your legs and fingers over, and repeat.

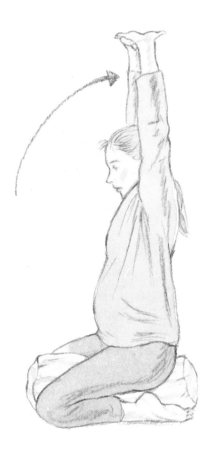

9 Reclining Tailor's pose

This pose, Supta Badha Konasana, opens up the abdominal area, stimulates pelvic circulation, releases tension in the hips and helps prepare the pelvic floor for childbirth.

Sit on the floor in the Tailor's pose (see page 60) with a support such as a cushion and beanbag firmly against your back. Lean back comfortably, without straining.

Press the soles of your feet together. To prevent your feet from slipping, loop a belt around your waist and feet. Rest your arms behind you, open the chest as you inhale, and concentrate on lifting the ribcage up and away from your abdomen.

Hold the position for as long as you wish.

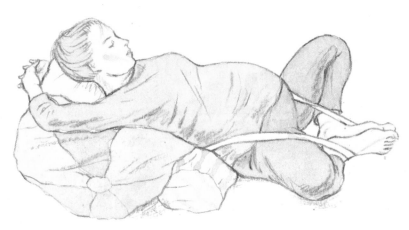

10 Supine pelvic tilt

This is similar to a standing pelvic tilt but more relaxing. You can use your increased body weight to assist the tilt.

Lie on your back, and bend your knees so that your feet are flat on the floor, hip-width apart, six inches from the buttocks.

Inhale, and on the exhalation, visualize lowering your baby very gently down towards your spine.

Press down with your feet, and feel your pelvis and back flattening into the earth.

Repeat two or three times.

Relax, lean your knees against one another and practise breath awareness (page 40).

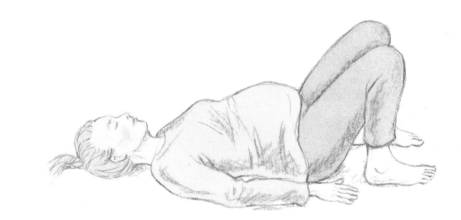

11 Arm extensions

These open up the shoulders (see page 42), relieving stiffness and encouraging a natural expansion of the breath.

Finish the sequence with the Body of Light exercise (see page 45)

Salute to the Earth – growing into gravity

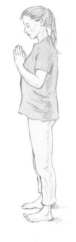

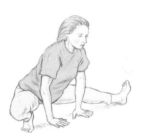

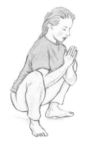

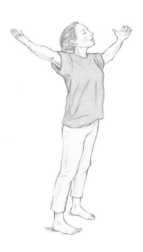

1 Mountain prayer and
17 Final Prayer

14 Half-squat

15 Touch the Earth

16 Heavenly stretch

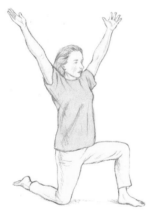

During pregnancy, your whole being will feel increasingly withdrawn to your pelvis, sacred cradle of your baby. In yogic terms, you are connecting with your root chakra, which is situated at the base of the body and connects with the earth via the legs. The root chakra is associated with survival and, in general, influences 'down-to-earth' matters. Pregnancy can make you feel part of the natural world and more 'earthed' than before.

13 Lift

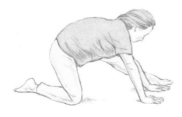

11 The Cat

10 The Sphinx

12 Rocking lunge

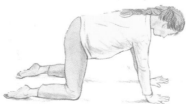

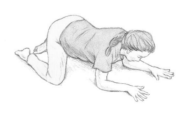

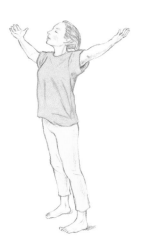

2 Heavenly stretch

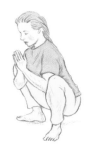

3 Touch the Earth

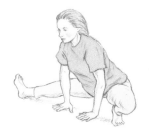

4 Half-squat

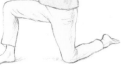

5 Lift

Rather than saluting the sun, a traditional yoga sequence of positions performed as one continuous exercise in preparation for the asanas, this continuous sequence acknowledges the nourishing and generous power of Mother Earth. It can be done at any time of day, round a square shape to represent the Earth, and begins and ends in the centre of your mat. Do it outdoors and smell the earth; do it indoors and feel the security of your surrounding walls.

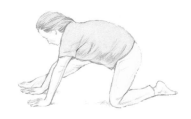

6 Rocking lunge

7 The Cat

9 The Sage's twist

8 The Thunderbolt

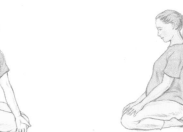

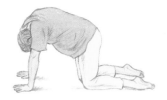

1 Mountain prayer

Stand in the centre of your mat, your feet hip-width apart.

With your hands in the prayer position, relax your shoulders and elbows down.

Silently greet the energy of the Earth by releasing your tailbone down, strengthening the legs and drawing your focus inwards to the centre of your being.

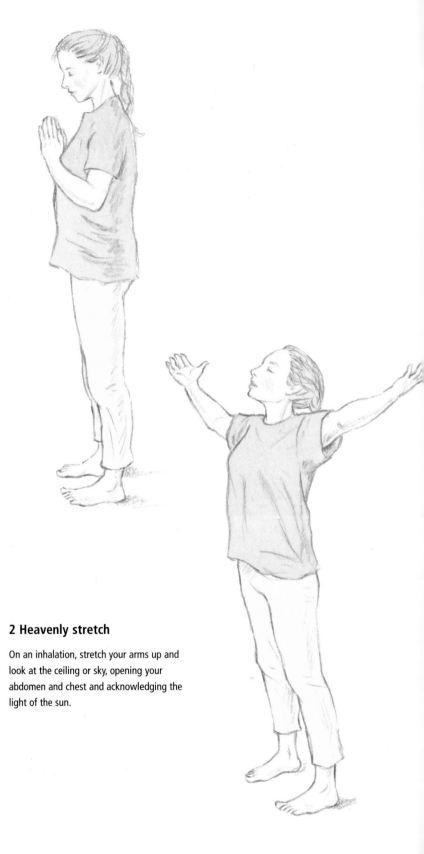

2 Heavenly stretch

On an inhalation, stretch your arms up and look at the ceiling or sky, opening your abdomen and chest and acknowledging the light of the sun.

3 Touch the Earth – squat

On the exhalation, drop down slowly into a squat. As you go down, turn your toes out slightly, keeping your heels hip-width apart.

With your hands in the prayer position again, gently ease your knees outwards with your elbows and feel your lower back moving downwards. Hold for at least 30 seconds.

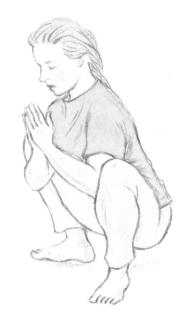

4 Half-squat

Still squatting, place your hands on the floor in front of you, slide your left leg out to the side and breathe into your left heel. You will come up on the toes of your right foot, so keep your hands on the floor. Hold the position for a couple of breaths.

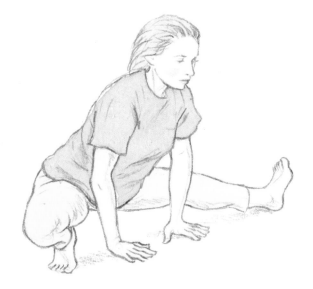

5 Lift

Keeping your hands on the floor, turn your left leg forward until it is kneeling on the floor. Step forward with your right foot and turn it out slightly.

Pressing firmly down with your right foot, breathe in, tucking the tailbone under so that your left thigh and torso are in line.

Lift your arms and open up the front of your body. Feel your inner sun shining.

You should feel stable as you lift up; if not, check your position with the illustration. Hold for two or three breaths.

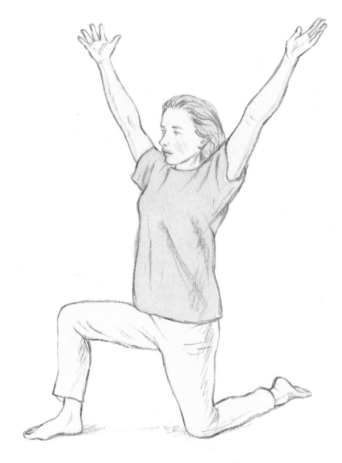

6 Rocking lunge

Come down as you exhale and bring your hands to the floor, shoulder-width apart, slightly in front of your left foot.

Take your right foot slightly forwards so that the outside of your right hand is parallel with the inside of your right foot.

Looking down at the space between your right foot and your hand, rock gently backwards and forwards, breathing easily and keeping your focus on your inner centre of gravity, wherever you perceive it to be.

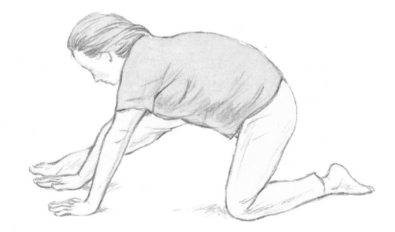

7 The Cat

Come to a still point and take your right leg back to the Cat position, so you are on all fours with your hands under your shoulders and your knees under your hips.

Open the palms of your hands and spread your fingers so that the middle fingers are parallel to one another.

Drop your head and relax your neck. Keeping your spine straight, release all the vertebrae in your neck.

As you exhale, tuck your tailbone under and draw your baby up to your spine, keeping the crown of your head released down.

Feel all your vertebrae separating one from another. On the inhalation release down to a straight-backed position, raising your head a little so that you are looking at the floor between your hands.

Repeat these movements twice more.

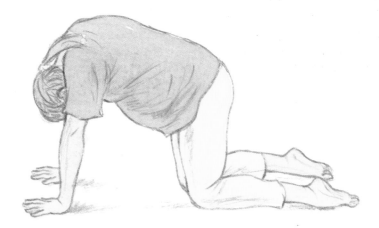

8 The Thunderbolt

Kneel with your thighs together and sit back on your heels. Sit on blocks or a cushion if necessary. If you are comfortable, move your feet apart and sit between them, keeping the thighs together.

Release your wrists, and be still for a moment, feeling your spine rooting down to the ground on the out-breath.

As you inhale, lift your spine without arching the back.

As you exhale, relax your shoulders downward.

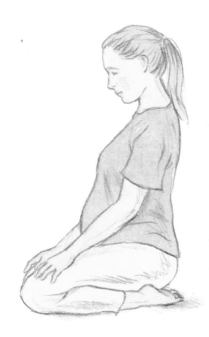

9 The Sage's twist

Take your hands to the floor to the right of your right thigh and simultaneously lift up your buttocks. Put a cushion or block under your right buttock so that your right heel is touching the outside of your left thigh and your left foot is crossing the right instep.

Tuck the fingers of your left hand under the outside of your right knee, so the palm of your hand is facing outwards. Place your right hand lightly on the floor or take it behind your back.

As you inhale, lift your spine. As you exhale, release a little and look over your right shoulder.

Your spine should be straight, with the energy gently spiralling up.

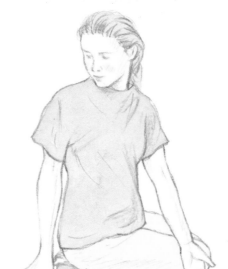

Keep your face and eyes soft. If they feel tense, go back a little and gently breathe into the resistance. Let the position ripen: don't force anything.

After 30 seconds, release back to the kneeling position and adjust so you are twisting to the other side. Repeat and return to the Thunderbolt.

10 The Sphinx

Widen your knees from the Cat position and lower your forearms and hands until they are flat on the floor and parallel with one another. Keep your head level with your spine.

As you exhale, continue to turn the tailbone under and lengthen the back of the neck. Release as you inhale. (The movement is similar to that of the Cat but more concentrated.)

Repeat twice more.

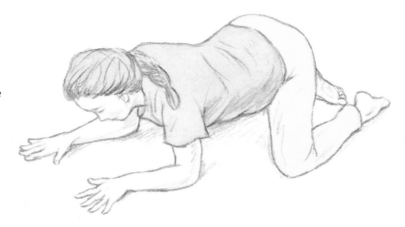

11 The Cat

Return to the Cat and flex the back for three breaths, as before.

12 Rocking lunge

Take your left foot to the outside of your left hand and lunge to the left, as before.

13 Lift

Take your left foot back slightly so it is flat on the floor and slightly turned out. Checking that you are stable, lift up on an inhalation, as before.

14 Half-squat

Returning your hands to the floor in front of you, tuck the toes of your left foot under, bring your right knee up off the floor and slide your left foot out to the side. Stretch into your left heel and lift with the sternum, but keep your hands on the floor.

15 Touch the Earth – squat

Withdraw your right heel and make sure you are stable. Sit comfortably in a squat for at least 30 seconds, as before.

16 Heavenly stretch

On an inhalation, rise up, using your thigh muscles and taking your arms out to the sides for balance. As you reach the upright position, bring your toes in so the outsides of your feet are parallel again. Lift your arms up to the heavens on an inhalation.

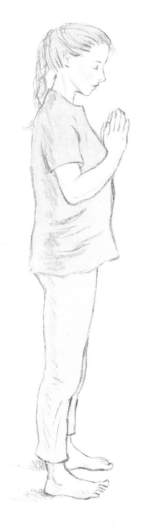

17 Final prayer

Return to your standing prayer position on the exhalation. Breathe quietly with relaxed shoulders, looking at the tips of your middle fingers, and return your attention to the centre of your being.

Tune in to your centre of gravity and remain centred. Repeat this sequence on the other side, taking the left leg out to the side first.

Finish with relaxation in the Corpse pose. See page 44.

Open to the light – a stronger stretch

This sequence develops the foundations laid in Touching base (page 51), and is also best done in the morning. The standing postures now grow roots and develop in self-confidence. Asanas become firm, but not rigid; like a strong mind, they need not be inflexible. These postures encourage introspection within movement, and help to deepen self-knowledge. They show that if you remain true to your nature you will never become uprooted.

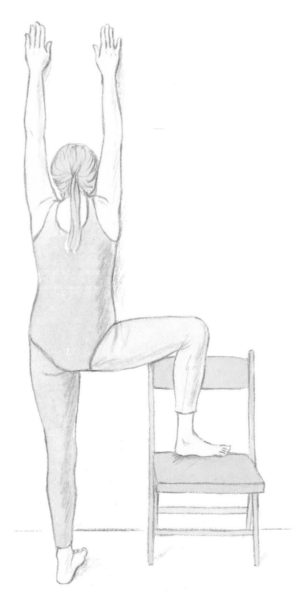

1 Step lunge

This position offers relief to the lower back and shoulders, opens up the hips and creates space in your abdomen for your growing baby. Use it also as a quick stretch on its own at any time.

Place a chair with its back close to the wall and stand slightly to the left of it, facing the wall so you are about eight inches away. Step your right foot up on to the seat of the chair, turning out the toes.

Raise your arms above your head and lean them against the wall. Lean forward from the base of your spine and rest your head on the wall.

Lean your chest against the wall and feel your shoulder blades flattening as you do so. As you exhale, feel the spine lengthening to the floor. Keep the supporting leg straight.

Hold for a minute, and repeat on the other side.

2 Growing a tree

This creates a connection between heaven and earth: while the feet are rooted to the ground, the upper body reaches towards the sky.

Standing firm and still, interlock the fingers and turn the palms away from you, straightening your elbows in front of you.

Inhale, and raise your arms above your head, stretching them back so that they are just behind your ears. Feel your armpits opening and the palms stretching to the ceiling. Flatten the shoulder blades and move the lower back downwards. Stand straight as a pine in a windless sky.

Inhale and, on the exhalation, swing your arms and upper body to the right. Keep your feet, legs and hips straight and grounded. Stretch the left arm and armpit and keep your head poised between your arms.

Do the same to the left.

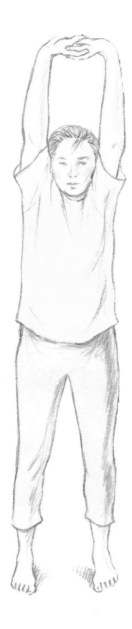
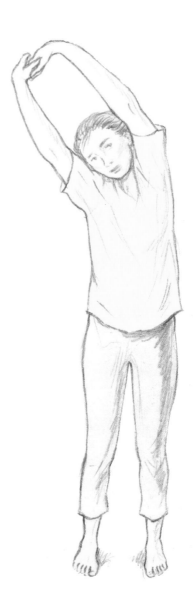

3 The Tree

If you are used to doing the Tree, you will be able to adapt to your increasing weight. To help you keep your balance, rest one hand on the back of a chair, as shown. This pose links earth and sky; it has poise, strength and equilibrium – like a tree.

Stand in the Mountain (page 53) and place the sole of one foot against the inside of the other thigh, as high as it will go. (If this is uncomfortable rest your foot on the opposite knee or on the seat of a chair.

On an inhalation, slowly raise one or both arms above your head, palms facing. Feel the armpits opening and the shoulder blades flattening as the twigs of your fingers stretch up to the light. Keep the tailbone turned under and the bent knee back.

Look straight ahead. Hold for up to 30 seconds and repeat on the other side.

4 The Mountain
See page 53.

5 First Warrior

The warrior poses are fighting poses, and the enemy is within: by slaying negative emotions the poses enhance concentration. They also strengthen the legs and lower back, improve balance, and open up the shoulders and abdomen. If you are not familiar with warrior poses, modify the stance or put a chair under the bent leg.

Caution: If you have low blood pressure, place your hands on your hips rather than raising them above your head.

Step your feet as wide apart as is comfortable. Turn the right foot out and the left foot in. Inhale, and raise the arms above the head, palms facing one another.

Rotate your hips and torso to the right. On the exhalation, breathe your left heel into the ground and, as you inhale, move the whole torso up and out of the pelvis. Imagine your lungs are helium balloons, anchored to the secure base of your stance but lifting you up and up.

(If your arms are tired, drop them and take a short rest before going on to the next step.)

Inhale, and drop the right thigh as far as it is comfortable, with the left leg fully stretched behind. Do not let the right knee swing sideways or overshoot the foot.

Bringing the palms of the hands together, gently arch the lower back, lift your head and look up at your hands.

Bring your weight back on to the left heel and use your breath to keep the torso light and lifted. Hold for no more than 30 seconds. Repeat on the left side.

6 The Cat with Mula Bandha

'Mula Bandha', meaning 'root lock', is the yogic interpretation of pelvic-floor exercises. It strengthens the pelvic floor and prevents the dissipation of downward-moving energy within the body, drawing it up to your baby. Do this exercise when you are familiar with synchronizing breath and movement in the Cat (see page 56).

On the exhalation, as you tuck your tailbone under, draw up the muscles of your pelvic floor. On the inhalation, as you straighten your back, release them.

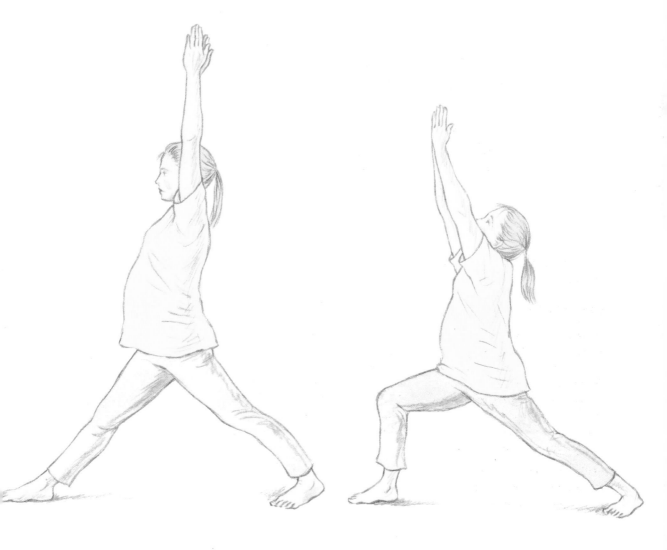

7 Extreme leg stretch

The head normally drops right down in this pose, but modify it in pregnancy by resting your head and arms on a support. The pose promotes pelvic circulation, relieves backache, opens the lungs and aids digestion.

Caution: Omit if you have high blood pressure, dizziness, breathlessness or abdominal pain, and if you have discomfort in the knees or lower back.

With a support about two feet in front of you, step your feet wide, the outsides of the feet parallel.

On an exhalation, slowly extend forward and down from the base of the spine, leading with the crown of the head, until you can rest your forearms on the support. Spread your toes and breathe your feet into the floor. Keep your legs straight.

Hold for at least 30 seconds, and for as long as you like.

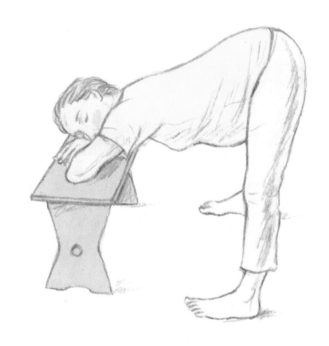

8 Triangle foot pose

This simple pose helps digestion, encourages pelvic circulation, relieves tired legs and is calming and refreshing. Use a belt to increase the stretch, and a support under the buttock if necessary.

Sit on the floor with your feet in front. Bend your right knee out to the side so your right calf is against the outside of your right thigh. The top of your foot should touch the floor and your toes point backwards. Keep your thighs together.

Loop a belt around your left foot and extend forwards on the exhalation, keeping your sternum open and the crown of your head leading the stretch. Maintain your centre of gravity in your right thigh.

Hold for two minutes and repeat on the other side.

9 Pelvic lift

This gives a good stretch to the lower back.

Caution: If the pose makes your thighs feel overstretched or lifts your knees, rest your elbows on a chair behind you.

Sit on the floor in the Thunderbolt position (see page 59). Place your hands flat on the floor six to eight inches behind you, shoulder-width apart.

Inhale, opening up the sternum and dropping the shoulders, and raise the buttocks from your feet. Tucking your tailbone under, feel a stretch from knees to sternum.

As you exhale, drop the buttocks back down to your heels.

Repeat twice, working with the breath.

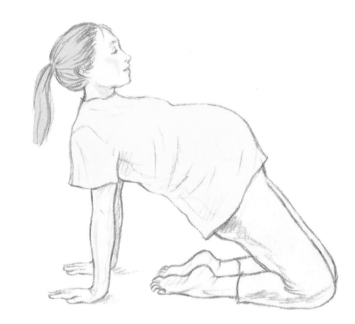

10 Supine back stretch and knee squeeze

This is a relaxing counterpoise to the pelvic lift, above.

Lie on your back in a pelvic tilt with the knees bent. On an inhalation, bring your right knee up over the side of your chest.

As you exhale, gently press on the knee to bring it farther down by your side and your lumbar spine to the floor. Be aware of each vertebra flattening against the floor. Breathing slowly and evenly, maintain the pose for as long as is comfortable.

Repeat with the other knee.

Roll on to your side and come up slowly.

11 Arm extensions
See page 42.

Finish the sequence with relaxation in the Corpse pose. See page 44.

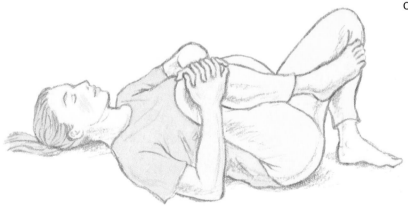

Heart of the sun – moving with energy

This is a more adventurous sequence, to be done in the morning when you have most energy. Omit pose numbers 1, 3 and 4 if you feel less energetic. Maintain your sense of inner calm and grow outwards from it, rather than over-extending to conform to an ideal. Use the modifications where necessary in order to enjoy the stretch without stress. Tension will be released from every part as you feel your sap rising.

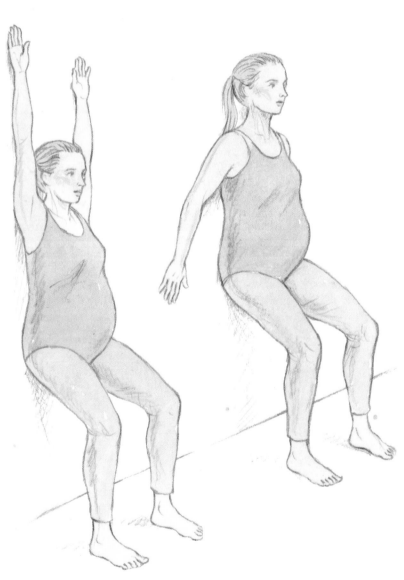

1 The phantom chair

This relieves strain in the lower back, opens the shoulders and strengthens the legs.

Stand with your back to a wall, heels 8–10 inches away. Flatten your whole back, including your shoulders, arms and the back of your head, to the wall. The middle of your back may not touch easily.

As you exhale, consciously relax your spine downwards. Bend your knees and slide slowly down the wall, tilting your pelvis so the middle vertebrae touch the wall.

Don't let your knees overreach your toes. You could also reach your arms up above your head, palms out, in this position.

Hold for as long as is comfortable, and then slide up again.

2 Upper back sideways stretch

This pose helps relieve aching in the shoulders, upper back and neck. As well as integrating it into your yoga practice, you can do this any time – seated at a desk or standing in the kitchen, for example.

Stand (or sit) comfortably with your back straight.

Put your right hand behind your back, palm outwards. Lift the elbow and slide the back of your hand up your back.

On an inhalation, raise the left arm, bent at the elbow, above your head.

On the exhalation, lean sideways to the right from the waist, gently curving your spine, neck, head and arm.

Hold the position for a few breaths, coming up slightly on an inhalation and going down again on the exhalation.

Repeat on the other side.

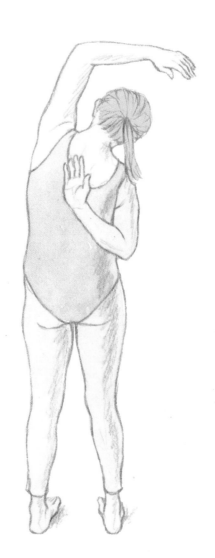

3 Strong standing side-stretch

This position gives each side of the body a long stretch, opens the shoulders and hips and strengthens the legs. Modify the pose by shortening your stance and using a chair under the thigh to support your weight.

Caution: To avoid stressing the sacro-iliac joint, take care to come out of the pose safely, as detailed below.

Step into a wide stance, and turn your right foot out to the right and your left foot in, as in the Triangle (page 54). Inhale, and raise your arms sideways until they are parallel to the ground, palms down.

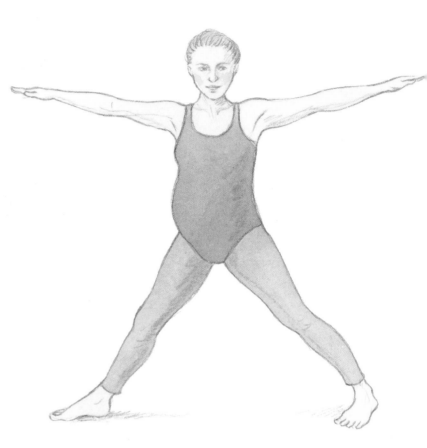

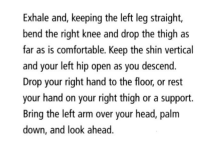

Exhale and, keeping the left leg straight, bend the right knee and drop the thigh as far as is comfortable. Keep the shin vertical and your left hip open as you descend. Drop your right hand to the floor, or rest your hand on your right thigh or a support. Bring the left arm over your head, palm down, and look ahead.

As you stretch, draw your weight back to the left heel. Feel the stretch all along your left side, from the heel to the fingertips. Hold for 20–30 seconds.

To come up, first raise the head and spine to vertical, and then step your feet back together. Repeat on the left side.

4 Second Warrior

Like the first Warrior (see page 78), this strong pose enhances concentration. It also stretches the legs and lower back and opens up the shoulders, abdomen and uterus.

Step your feet wide and turn the left foot out and the right foot in.

Raise the arms sideways, palms down. Turn and look along your left arm and feel your right hip opening. Turn the tailbone under and lengthen your back.

As you inhale, feel the breath coming up your spine, dividing at the shoulder blades and reaching along your arms, buoying them up.

As you exhale, slowly bend your left knee, but keep your spine vertical as you descend. If this feels strenuous, use a chair.

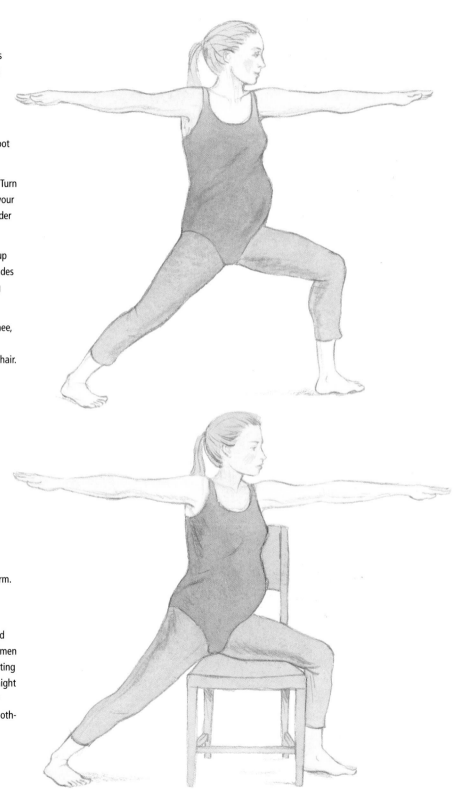

Turn your head to look along the left arm. Keep your neck soft and don't tilt your head forward.

Keep the right heel firmly on the ground and the right leg straight. Lift the abdomen up and away from the pelvic floor, creating space for the baby. Keep your back straight and breathe into the pose, feeling your arms stretching ever away from one another. Hold for a maximum of 20 seconds.

Repeat on the other side.

5 Resting position

This position helps you catch your breath and regain your sense of centredness between the stronger standing poses. Place a pillow on the back of the chair to soften it.

Sit astride a chair, facing the back.

Rest your head on your folded arms and release from your lower back.

Breathe easily.

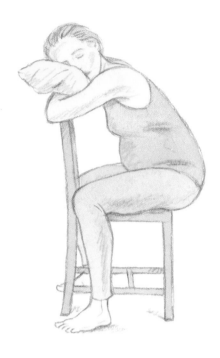

6 Swinging low

This stretching and twisting of the lumbar vertebrae relieve backache. Later in the pregnancy, widen your stance and don't stretch downward, just sideways.

Stand with your feet straight and hip-width apart. Fold your arms and grasp the opposite elbow with each hand. Bend forward from the waist, looking over your arms. Pin the heels down, spread the toes and keep the legs straight. Stretch your sternum forward, opening up the chest and lumbar vertebrae. Swing to the right until your forearms are parallel to the outside of the right foot.

On the exhalation, extend your elbows down. Keep both legs straight and vertical, allowing the lumbar vertebrae to twist. Do not lean further down than is comfortable, and don't hold for more than a couple of breaths. Repeat on the other side.

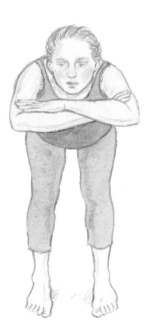

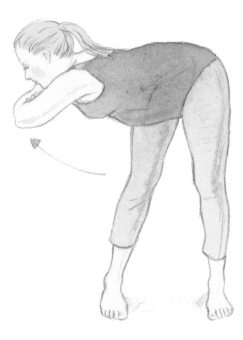

7 Three-legged Cat

This pose helps open and loosen the hip joints.

Go into the Cat (page 56) and, with your back straight, drop down on to your left forearm and raise your right leg.

Keeping the knee bent, rotate the leg from the hip, two or three times in each direction.

Repeat with the left leg.

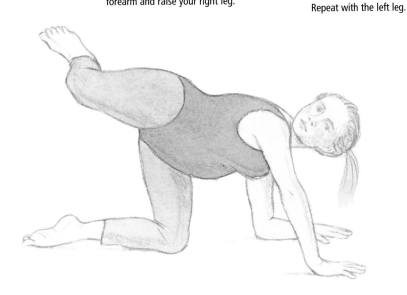

8 Supine against a wall

This pose counterbalances the more active asanas of this sequence.

Prepare as described on page 62, starting with your legs straight up.

With breath awareness, and when you feel ready, allow your feet to slide slowly apart down the wall, as shown on page 62. Do not push or strain – leave it to gravity. Allow your hips to relax as you exhale, and hold for as long as is comfortable.

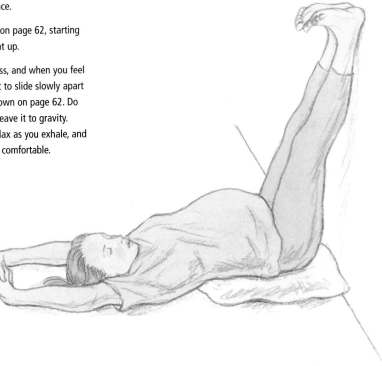

9 Knee circles

This moving pose counters the previous static asana and helps you prepare for squatting by increasing flexibility in your hips.

Still supine, bend your knees and bring them to either side of your chest.

Make circles in the air with your knees, so that you feel your pelvis describing circles on the floor.

Repeat in the other direction.

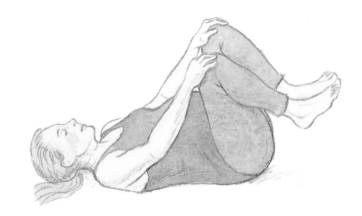

10 Squat

See also pages 57 and 71. Breathe out at length through the mouth with puckered lips, and in through the nose.

Caution: If you are in the last eight weeks of pregnancy and your baby is in the breech position, avoid squatting.

Drop down into a squat, and to extend the pose try one of the following variants:

Arms behind your back

Holding on to the back of a chair

With your back to a wall (not shown)

11 Seated angle pose
See page 58.

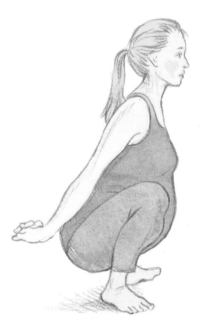

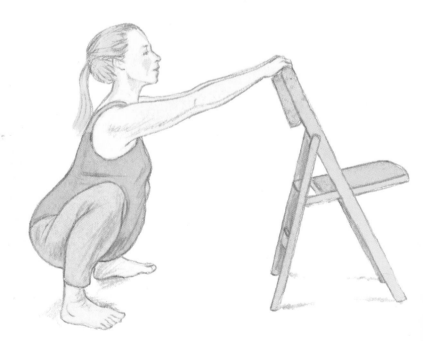

12 Lion pose

This relieves tension in the eyes, throat, neck and face. It also clears the throat chakra and is a good preparation for making sounds during labour.

Sit or kneel in any comfortable position. Stretch your hands out and place them either on the floor or on your knees.

Take a deep inhalation. On the exhalation, lean forward on your hands and open your eyes and mouth wide and, sticking your tongue out as far as it will go, roar from deep in your abdomen. Repeat three times.

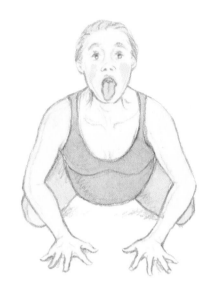

13 Magical pose

Simple though it seems, this is one of the most beneficial yoga positions. Both relaxing and exhilarating, it stimulates blood flow in the pelvis, stretching and strengthening the pelvic floor. The spine, remaining upright, conducts energy to the brain. Use cushions under the knees if necessary.

Sit with your spine erect and legs outstretched. Bend your right knee and cradle your right ankle with your hands. Relax the whole leg, and gently swing it so the knee describes an arc and you feel the hip moving in its socket. Repeat with the left leg.

Place your right heel up by the perineum, the sole of the foot against the inner left thigh. Place the left foot on top of the right, with the heel facing upwards and the ball of the foot tucked between the calf and thigh of the right leg. Hold for as long as you like.

Finish the sequence with breathing and relaxation in the Corpse pose.

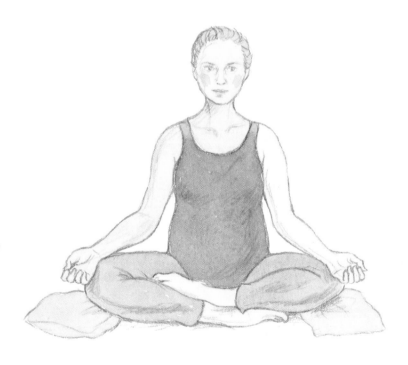

Learning to fly – from gravity to levity

This sequence may be done at any time of day, whenever you have time to give it your full attention. A delicious stretch to the whole back is combined with asanas to improve the circulation in the legs, flex the wrists and open the shoulders. You will find yourself shedding 'baggage', and the result is a feeling of levity, as if you could fly. Do pose numbers 7 and 11 only if you are already used to them.

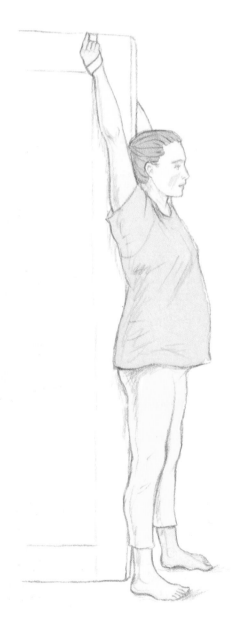

1 Back stretch with a door

This pose uses the edge of a door and a belt to stretch the back, and is also a good supported shoulder opener that does not strain the spine. If you keep a belt permanently looped over a door, you can have a stretch whenever you go past.

Loop a belt over the top of a door and, with your back to the door, reach your hands up so they are stretched (if you can reach without a belt, just clasp the top of the door).

As you exhale, turn your tailbone under and feel the edge of the door along the length of your back.

Keep your legs straight and your armpits open. Do for as long as is comfortable.

2 Simple lunge

This position, which is illustrated on page 52, lengthens the lower back, encouraging the tailbone to turn under, and also opens the shoulders and flexes the heels for easier squatting.

Stand facing a wall, toes 8–12 inches away from it. Step one foot back about two feet, bend the leading knee and keep the back leg straight, with both heels on the floor. Toes and hips face forwards.

Lean your forearms against the wall and rest your head on the wall below so that your forehead and elbows are in line.

As you exhale, feel the calf and heels of the back leg lengthening. Hold for a minute, breathing easily. Repeat on the other side.

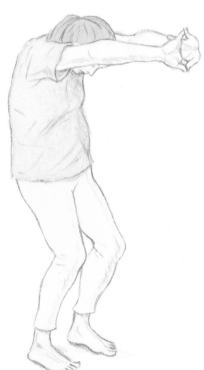

3 Shoulder blade fan

This exercise helps release tension in the middle of the shoulders. (It is quick and easy to do in any spare moment.)

Standing with your feet hip-width apart, interlock your fingers and, as you exhale, extend them away from you. At the same time bend your knees and bring your head between your arms.

As you inhale, bend your elbows and bring your hands to your sternum, straightening your legs and spine as you do so.

On your next inhalation, separate your hands and draw your elbows back, squeezing the shoulder blades together. Don't raise the shoulders or arch your back. Repeat three times, and relax.

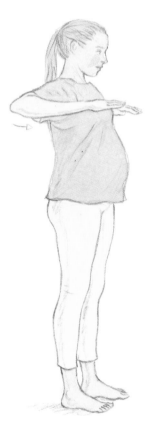

4 Standing forward bend

See page 55.

5 Elbow circles

This releases congestion in the shoulders. Return to a sitting position and place your hands on your shoulders.

Inhale, and breathe comfortably and deeply as you describe circles in the air with your elbows. Make circles both from front to back and back to front, moving both elbows in unison. Repeat several times each way.

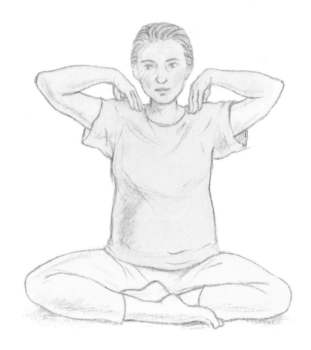

6 Cow-head pose

Part 1 of this pose stretches the outside of your hip joints and helps relieve discomfort in the sacro-iliac joints. If you find it strains your knees, however, do part 2 only, in any position. Part 2 opens up the shoulders.

Part 1

Go into the Cat (page 56), then cross your right leg in front of your left. Swing your left foot out to the side, and slowly sit back on the floor between your feet.

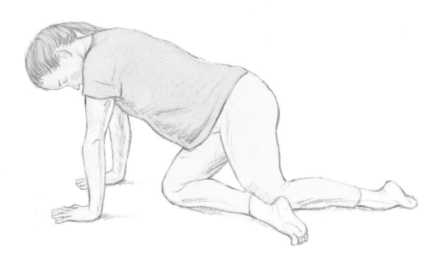

Align your knees so they are now positioned one on top of the other.

Rest your hands on top of your knees and
relax, breathing evenly. Hold for as long as
is comfortable and repeat on the other side.

Modifications: If you cannot sit between
your feet, sit either on the lower leg or on a
block placed beside the heel of the lower
foot. If you cannot sit comfortably in this
position, sit in either Thunderbolt or any
other comfortable position for part 2.

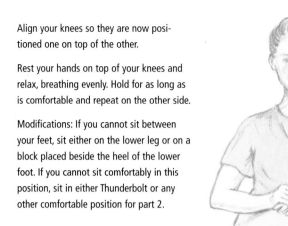

Part 2

Raise your right elbow vertically above your
head and drop the right hand down behind
you and catch the fingers of the left hand.
Keep the right upper arm close to the head
and the elbow up.

Move the shoulder blades in. Avoid arching
your back by breathing down into your tailbone on the out-breath. Look ahead, keeping your eyes, face and neck relaxed.

If your hands do not reach each other, sus-
pend a belt or scarf from your right hand
and catch it with the left. Hold for 30
seconds and repeat on the other side.

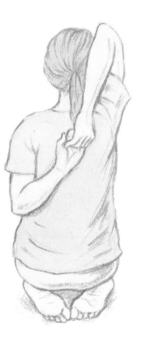
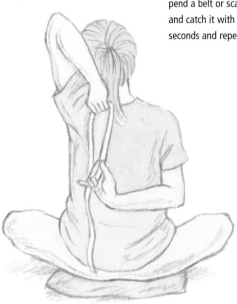

7 All-round extension

This exercise releases the lower back and opens up the sternum and shoulders, flexing the entire spine.

Stand in front of a ledge or chair-back and step your left foot back a comfortable distance so that both feet face the support. Keep your hips in line with each another. (If they are out of line, come up on the toes of your left foot and release your left hip forwards before taking the left heel back to the floor.)

Put your hands on your hips.

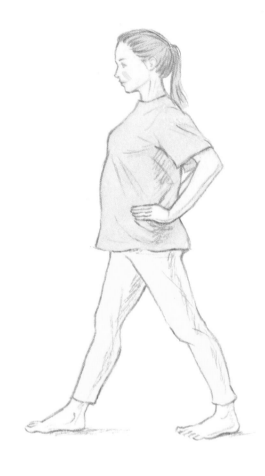

Inhale, and bring your elbows back, squeezing your shoulder blades together. On the exhalation, stretch your arms and spine forward and rest your hands lightly on the support. Keep your legs at equal angles, that is, don't have one more upright than the other. Lead the stretch with your sternum, and move the crown of your head and your arms forward on the exhalation.

Repeat on the left side.

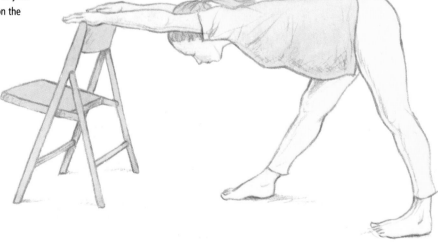

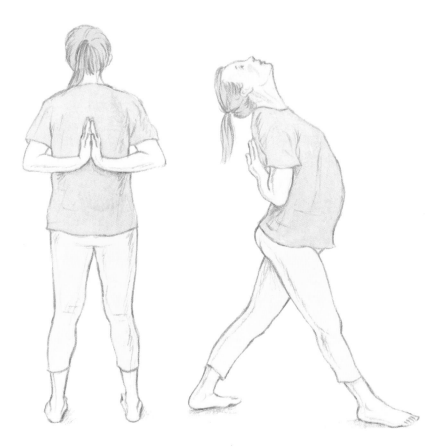

Stand in the Mountain pose (see page 53). Inhale, bring your hands behind your back and, if you can, place your palms together in the prayer position. Move your elbows back to press your hands together. If this is difficult, simply clasp your hands or fold your arms. Step one foot back a comfortable distance.

Inhale, and on the exhalation, bend backward slightly from the waist, but do not strain. Lead the stretch with the sternum. Look up and breathe evenly. Repeat on the other side.

8 Supine back stretch and knee squeeze
See page 81.

9 Neck loosener

As with all the neck exercises, this releases tension from the head, neck and shoulders. Sit straight up in any comfortable position, inhale, and on the exhalation turn your neck to the right, keeping the head upright and the spine vertical.

As you inhale, bring the head halfway back to the centre. Again, turn your head to the right, and exhale through trumpet-shaped lips, making a small 'hoo' ing sound. Let your neck twist with the breath and do not force it; you will find that you go a little further each time. Repeat three times and do the same on the left side.

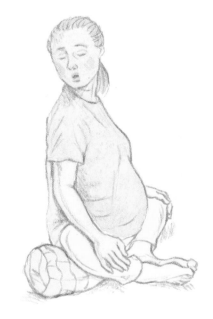

10 Simple supine twist

Supine twists gently separate the vertebrae of the lower back and relieve backache. They also stimulate blood flow here and in other key areas of tension – inner thighs, neck and shoulders,

Lie on your back with your knees bent and your feet flat on the ground, hip-width apart. Stretch your arms out to the sides, palms down. Flatten your whole spine, including the back of the neck, to the floor.

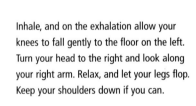

Inhale, and on the exhalation allow your knees to fall gently to the floor on the left. Turn your head to the right and look along your right arm. Relax, and let your legs flop. Keep your shoulders down if you can.

Hold the position for 30 seconds, breathing normally. Repeat on the other side.

11 Full Lotus

If you cannot do the full Lotus, try the less strenuous half Lotus, opposite. In each case place a rolled blanket or cushion under the left knee if you need support.

Sit on the floor and flex your legs as for the Magical pose (page 89). Supporting your right leg with the left hand, thread your right arm through the crook of your bent knee and gently draw it back, moving the flesh of the right calf as you do so. This will give your knee more space.

Slowly bring your right heel across to the left thigh, as far as it will comfortably go, and rest the back of the foot there. Place the heel of the left foot as far up and across the right thigh, as is comfortable.

Rest your hands on your knees, raise the torso and feel the lumbar vertebrae separating. Raise your sternum, drop the shoulders and don't puff out the chest. Look down or straight ahead and breathe gently. Maintain for as long as you like.

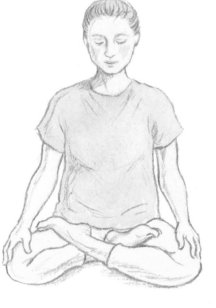

Half Lotus

This is a less strenuous form of the Lotus position. In the later months of pregnancy, modify the pose by sitting on a block, cushion, small stool, bolster or beanbag.

Sit on the floor and position your right leg and foot as for the Lotus, but just tuck your left foot under your right leg.

Rest your hands on your knees, stretch the spine vertically and feel the lumbar vertebrae separating. Raise your sternum, drop the shoulders and don't puff out the chest.

Hold for as long as you like. If you get pins and needles, change legs immediately.

Finish this sequence with Bee breath (see page 108), followed by Tratak (below) and relaxation in the Corpse pose.

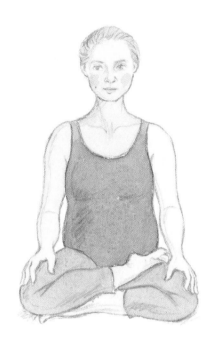

Tratak – candle gazing

The practice of Tratak involves gazing at a fixed object such as a candle, and is a simple way of relaxing the eyes and encouraging concentration. This does not mean concentration in the sense of tensing the muscles as we seek to exclude all distractions, but rather an all-embracing absorption of the body, mind and emotions. Even the eye muscles are relaxed but focused.

Tratak is a practical tool for aiding visualization, and as such is a step towards meditation. You can do Tratak after Pranayama; see page 106. Always follow Tratak with visualization and/or relaxation.

Caution: If a candle causes spots before the eyes, use a flower or any other small, pleasing object. If you wear hard contact lenses or suffer from a detached retina, keep blinking. If you wear glasses it is better to remove them for these exercises, as glasses condition the eye muscles to a particular focus, which Tratak seeks to soften.

Position a candle two to three feet away from you, with the flame at eye level. The flame must be still – if it flickers, eliminate the source of the draught.

Sit in a relaxed, comfortable position, with a straight spine. Look at the brightest part of the flame. Try not to blink, but never mind if you do. Absorb the softness of the bright flame into your eyes and your whole body.

After a couple of minutes, bring the palms of your hands over your eyes with your fingers on your forehead and, keeping your eyes open, gaze into the darkness.

After 30 seconds close your eyes and, if you see the image of the flame, bring it up to your forehead. Feel the light suffusing through your forehead and whole body.

Repeat once or twice more. On the final palming, rub your hands briskly together before you bring them up over your eyes.

Shining star – a stretch from the centre

Just as a star radiates light, this sequence works on stretching your body out in all directions from a central point: your baby. It opens the hips, strengthens the legs, lifts the abdomen and lungs, lengthens the arms and, with the Half-moon pose, provides dynamic relief to the pelvic floor. Circulation is stimulated and you will feel light and open. This is a daytime routine that, by omitting poses 6 and 7, adapts to evening use. Omit these two poses and number 12 if you are not already able in them, whatever the time of day. Remember: always stretch from the centre.

1 Arm extensions in a supine pelvic tilt
See page 67.

2 Leg extensions

This is a relaxing way of simultaneously opening up your hips and stretching your hamstrings prior to doing standing positions.

Lie on your back as for the pelvic tilt, above. Lift your right foot and catch it with your right hand, or with a belt or scarf. Raise the leg vertically above you and hold it there for up to a minute, keeping the left shoulder flat to the ground or a support.

Repeat with the left leg.

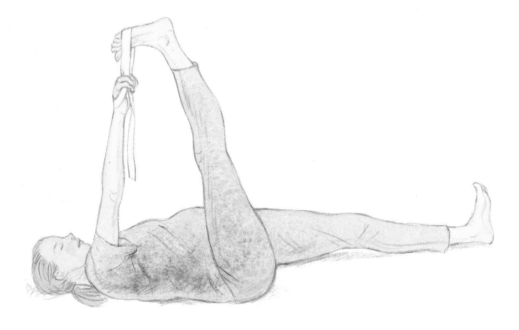

3 Sideways hip release

The more hip openers are practised before-hand, the easier it will be to open the hips during the birth process. Hip openers aid pelvic circulation, which benefits you and the baby. They also tone the pelvic floor and release any tension there. They can be useful in late pregnancy, when the pubic joint is loosening and perhaps causing discomfort.

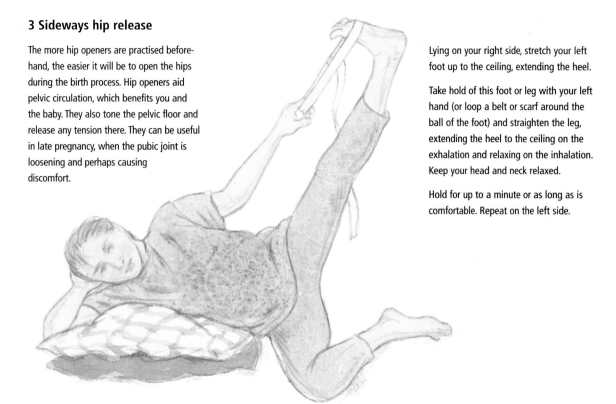

Lying on your right side, stretch your left foot up to the ceiling, extending the heel.

Take hold of this foot or leg with your left hand (or loop a belt or scarf around the ball of the foot) and straighten the leg, extending the heel to the ceiling on the exhalation and relaxing on the inhalation. Keep your head and neck relaxed.

Hold for up to a minute or as long as is comfortable. Repeat on the left side.

4 Extended Cat

This gives a wonderful feeling of length. Extending opposite parts of the body also helps with co-ordination and balance.

Go into the Cat (page 56) and, keeping the back straight but raising the head slightly, lift the right arm and extend it in front of you, palm down.

Raise the left leg and extend the heel out behind you. Hold for 30 seconds, breathing evenly. Repeat on the other side.

5 The Triangle
See page 54.

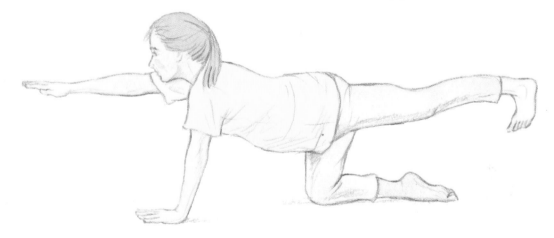

6 Half-moon

Do this pose against a wall for support. Although it looks strenuous, if your centre of gravity is secure the pose can be surprisingly light. It helps balance, strengthens the legs, opens the shoulders and hips, provides dynamic relief to the pelvic floor, and helps you open up to your 'inner light'.

Caution: If you have not done this pose before, do not begin it later than the start of the second trimester. This allows you to adapt to your changing weight.

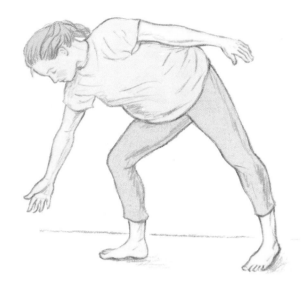

Have a wide stretch of wall clear and stand with your back to it, your heels a few inches away. Step your feet comfortably apart, as for the Triangle (page 54), and turn the right foot out and the left foot in. Inhale, and raise the arms to the sides, palms down.

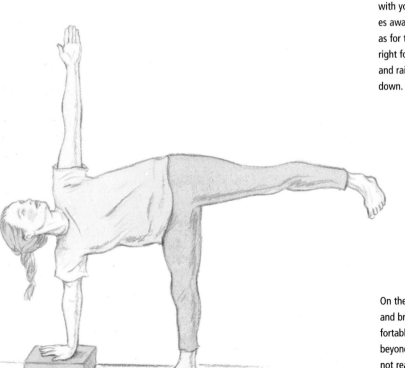

On the next exhalation, bend the right knee and bring your right hand down to a comfortable point on the floor just behind and beyond the right foot. If your hand does not reach the floor comfortably, use a support such as books or a low stool.

Simultaneously straighten the right leg and raise your left leg until it is parallel with the ground.

Raise the left arm, open your chest and look straight ahead. Lead the stretch of your spine with the crown of your head. If you are able, slowly turn your head and look up at your left hand.

Extend the left heel away from you, toes pointing down. Put your mind into the supporting leg; if you have that balance, the rest will follow. Separate your shoulder blades and feel very open. Hold for 20 seconds.

Repeat on the left side.

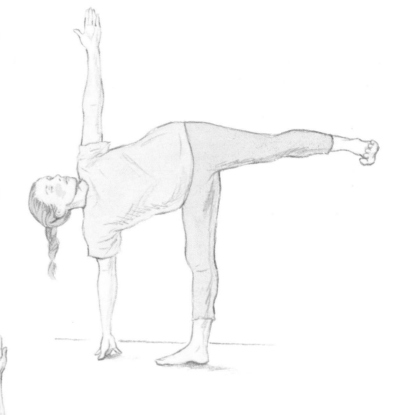

7 Reverse Triangle using a chair

This position gives a gentle twist to the lower back, opens up the shoulders and strengthens the legs and feet. Stand in the Triangle stance (see 5 above), right foot out and left foot in, and raise your arms. Look along your left arm.

Inhale, and rotate your arms, following your left hand with your eyes. Rest your left hand lightly on your support and stretch your right hand up to the sky.

Be strong with the left leg and foot and feel the gentle twist on your lower back and the opening between your shoulder blades. Hold for no longer than 20 seconds and gracefully return.

8 The Cat
See page 56.

9 Sideways stretch

The benefits of this stretch are the same as for the seated angle pose on page 58, but, because one leg is folded in, it is slightly easier. The sideways movement gives an excellent lateral stretch to the spine.

Caution: Do not overstretch. If you can't reach your toes, use a belt or scarf.

From the seated angle pose, tuck your right leg in and slide your left hand, palm facing outwards, along your left leg. Extend to the left. Keep your neck loose with the crown of your head leading the stretch and your right buttock on the ground.

If you can reach, grasp the toes of your left foot, or use a belt looped around the ball of the foot. Inhale, and raise your right arm. Exhale, and bring it over your head, bending the elbow. Hold for 30 seconds or so, breathing evenly.

Come up slowly and repeat on the other side.

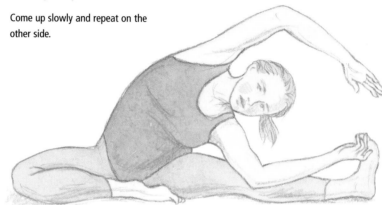

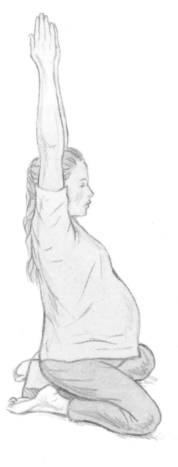

10 Seated wall lunge

This opens up the shoulders, hips and lower back in a peaceful, resting way. Sit on a low stool or a block in the later months.

Kneel about six inches away from and facing a wall. Widen your knees so they are well apart and you are sitting on your lower legs and heels.

On an inhalation, bring your arms up above your head. As you exhale, bring the palms of your hands and forearms flat against the wall. Relax forward into the wall.

Turn your tailbone under and feel your pelvis sinking down toward the floor as your upper back and arms lift up. Feel your shoulders opening.

Relax and hold for a few breaths.

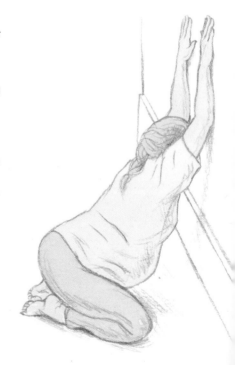

11 Supine twist (Universal pose)

Twists improve the circulation to the spine and release tension, thus reducing stress and irritability.

Lying flat on your back, bend your right knee so that your heel touches the buttock. Exhale, and flatten your entire spine, including the back of the neck, to the floor.

Spread your arms out to the sides, releasing your palms to the floor.

Inhale, and on the exhalation simultaneously bring your right knee down toward the floor on the left side and turn your head to the right.

With your left hand, draw the knee gently toward the floor. (Support the knee with a cushion if it does not reach.) As you inhale, feel the centre of your back opening. Hold for no more than 30 seconds.

Repeat on the left side.

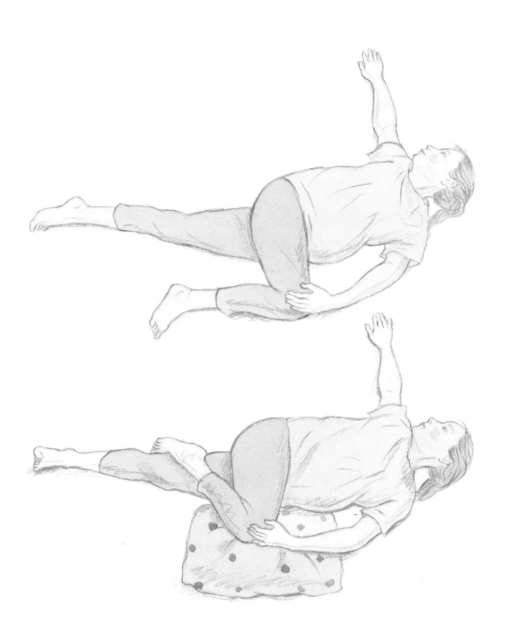

12 Reclining Thunderbolt

This pose, Supta Virasana, can be done at all times, even after meals. It stimulates blood flow in the pelvic region and the digestive tract, dispelling constipation, nausea and flatulence. It opens up the lungs and provides space for the growing baby and relaxation for you. It also revives tired legs. Arrange support beforehand, such as a block, cushion or beanbag.

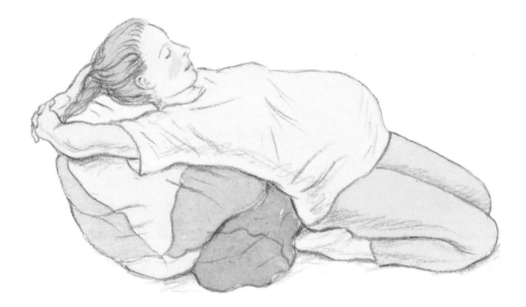

Caution: Omit this pose if you have high blood pressure or varicose veins, unless you have adequate support (that allows the free blood circulation under the buttocks and thighs). If your knees rise up as you lean back, come up at once. Either use higher support or substitute the reclining Tailor's pose (page 66).

Sit in the Thunderbolt pose (see page 59) with your support behind you.

Lean back on your right elbow and forearm and, without using your abdominal muscles, slowly bring your weight back on to the support. Make sure you are firmly propped at your lower back, shoulders and head.

Bring your arms back over your head, and rest them behind you or, if this is uncomfortable, by your sides. Lift your sternum, tuck your chin down and open up your armpits. Keep your thighs and knees together.

Maintain the pose for as long as you wish.

13 Neck circles

This stretching exercise, done in one continuous movement, relieves tension in the neck and shoulder muscles.

Caution: Do only small circles If you have low blood pressure, since moving the head around may cause dizziness.

Sit in the half Lotus (page 97) with your hands on your knees. Stretch your spine upwards, and keep it vertical throughout. Inhale, and as you do so, slowly turn your head to the right, stretching but not overstretching, over the right shoulder, and then tilt it gently backwards.

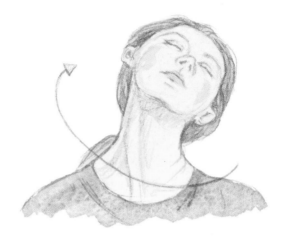

Keeping your head tilted back and exhaling, slowly move your head to the left until you are looking over your left shoulder, and then face forward again. By the time you have completed a full breath, the top of your head has described a complete circle.

Repeat twice in each direction.

14 Alternate nostril breathing
See page 109.

15 Om
See page 111.

Finish the sequence with relaxation in the Corpse pose.

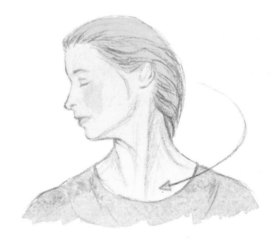

Pranayama: control of the breath

The Sanskrit word 'Pranayama' signifies control, not just of the breath, but of prana – the life force itself. Regular Pranayama practice will increase your body's vitality, boost your immune system and create inner calm. By cultivating breathing patterns while you are pregnant, you can control anxiety, insomnia and lethargy. You will also find that in labour the breath will come of its own accord, producing a state of altered consciousness not unlike deep meditation. It will help you stay calm and relaxed, increase the supply of oxygen to you and the baby, and make delivery easier.

Pranayama is usually done after asanas, since the ultimate aim of flexing and strengthening the body is to be able to sit still comfortably in order to follow the higher practices of yoga. These include Pranayama as well as sense withdrawal, concentration, meditation and absorption. You can, however, practise Pranayama at any time, as long as you are in a quiet and appropriate environment. Choose any of the breaths described in this section, although some are more suitable for certain times of the day than others. For example, intuitive breath is good first thing in the morning, as it is quite strong and invigorating. The alternate nostril breath and the Bee breath are useful at the end of the day, especially if you have difficulty sleeping. These breaths encourage inner calm and harmony by triggering the relaxation response, and you will find that sleep comes more easily.

Pranayama in practice

If you have never done Pranayama before, ensure that you are thoroughly used to the breath awareness exercises detailed in chapter 3, Yoga for the first trimester. It is not necessary to do more than one Pranayama exercise per session, but if you feel comfortable you may wish to do more, especially in the last trimester. However, always leave time for relaxation afterwards. Read the instructions carefully and take things slowly. Practised well, breath control is the key to self-control.

If you are used to Pranayama, Anuloma Viloma is a lovely breath that you can practise at any time as long as you do not suffer from low blood pressure. If you are not familiar with this, the simple version of alternate nostril breathing (page 109) is sufficient.

Pranayama is a shy and subtle friend. Treat it harshly and you will only reinforce established patterns. Treated with respect and sensitivity, however, it will open up the tender leaves curled at the centre of your being. Be open and gentle in your practice and the gifts of Pranayama will bless you.

Intuitive breath

This breath is known as Ujaiyi Pranayama in Sanskrit. The word 'Ujaiyi' literally means 'victorious'. This breath draws energy upwards and vanquishes negative thoughts, replacing them with feelings of tranquillity and intuition.

It involves contracting the muscles in the throat to produce a soft, silvery hissing sound. This naturally lengthens the out-breath, which has a calming effect that is also invigorating. It is reputed to banish phlegm, the root of all disease, and to strengthen the nervous and digestive systems. It is especially beneficial to people with low blood pressure, low energy, scattered thoughts or a weak heart.

Caution: Over-constriction of the throat can cause a roaring sound and create tension in the head, so keep the pressure moderate. If you have high blood pressure, take extra care to elongate the out-breath and not to hold it. If at any time the breathing becomes too 'muscular', revert to normal breathing. If you get pins and needles or cramp, change your position.

Sit in any comfortable position with your hands in your lap or on your knees, and close your eyes. As you breathe in, open up your sternum, and feel the breath gently filling your lungs. As you breathe out, melt your shoulders downwards and, slowly and carefully, empty your lungs.

Soften the neck muscles, let your tongue lie softly at the bottom of your mouth and feel your face lighten.

Breathe easily and normally for a few minutes. Keep your attention fully on your breath, your spine lifting but not rigid, and relax your abdomen so that it is soft.

Now lengthen the breaths by constricting the muscles of the glottis, that is, the muscles at the top of the larynx, to create a soft, silvery, hissing sound. Do this for two minutes, and return to normal breathing.

Gradually extend the length of time you do Ujaiyi until you can do it for five minutes. When you are comfortable with Ujaiyi breathing you can add a silent, simple mantra. As you breathe in, repeat to yourself 'Soh'. As you breathe out, repeat to yourself `Hum'. (Soh Hum: 'I am that'.)

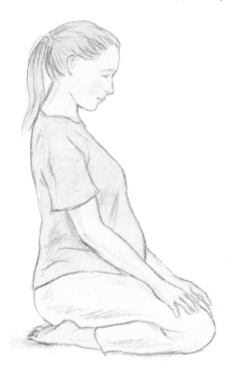

Spacious breath

In the later months of pregnancy, your breathing may feel constricted as your baby pushes up into your lungs, and the abdomen may even bulge over the lower ribs. The spacious breath helps to create space between you and your baby. You can do it sitting upright, but it is best (unless you are in labour) to do it lying back in a reclining Tailor's pose.

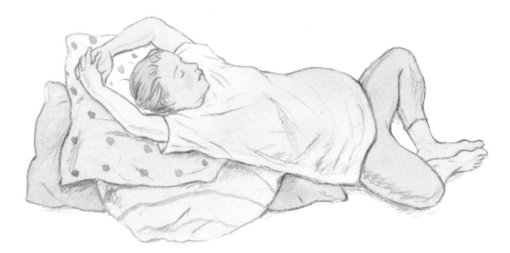

If you do this breath daily, you will be able to draw on it automatically during labour. It will give you a good oxygen supply, alleviate weight from the uterus and provide some pain relief.

As you inhale, roll your shoulders back and draw the air softly down to the bottom of your lungs, so they come up and off the belly. Allow your lower ribs to 'fly' open and away from your baby.

Exhale at length, feeling your lungs gently touching back to your baby. Don't let the abdomen 'overtake' the lungs. Repeat up to 10 times, with the out-breath longer than the in-breath.

Bee breath

In this breath (Bhramari) you make the sound of a bee humming, which is amplified by closing your ears. It has a direct impact on the pituitary gland, which influences the relaxation response. Regular practice of this will reduce blood pressure and induce calm confidence.

Caution: Omit this if it makes you dizzy.

Sit on a low stool with your feet apart and flat on the ground, elbows on your knees. Bend your head forward slightly, and place your thumbs in or over your ears.

Inhale, and on the exhalation, make a soft humming sound like a bee. If you take your thumbs momentarily away the humming will be soft; inside your head with your ears blocked, however, it will be quite loud.

Let the breath come out smoothly, and imagine you are a bee, flying purposefully from flower to flower. Inhale without sound, and repeat eight more times. This is one round. Breathe easily, and build up gradually to five rounds.

Alternate nostril breathing

In this exercise (Nadi Sodhana) you breathe alternately through each nostril. This balances the subtle energies of the body and induces calm and relaxation. Though it may seem awkward to do at first, it will come easily once you are used to it. It acts as a natural sedative and is safe and effective for counteracting insomnia, especially in the last month of pregnancy. If, as is common during pregnancy, one nostril is blocked, drain it before you begin by lying down on the opposite side to the congestion for a few minutes, or do Neti (page 110).

Sit comfortably, and either fold down the index and middle fingers of your right hand so they rest lightly on your palm, or stretch them out straight and rest them on your forehead.

Place your thumb lightly on your right nostril and your ring and little fingers on your left nostril – without restricting breathing – so that your fingertips rest in the indentations at the sides of your nostrils.

Breathing normally, practise applying gentle pressure on alternate sides, so one nostril at a time is closed. With both nostrils free, inhale deeply.

Without holding your breath at any stage, compress the right nostril with your thumb and exhale evenly through your left nostril.

Inhale through your left nostril. When your lungs are full, and without holding your breath, smoothly change over so your thumb lifts up and your ring and little finger compress the left nostril.

Exhale and inhale through the right nostril before changing over again. Exhale and inhale through the left nostril and change fingers. Keep the breaths smooth, even and of equal length. Repeat this cycle until you have done four cycles, and rest.

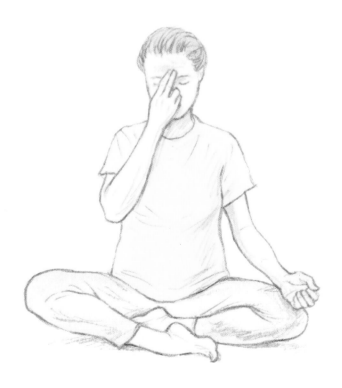

Mudra

A mudra is a gesture that aligns the meridians (energy channels) of the subtle body. You may find that holding your hands in different positions during breathing exercises creates subtle changes in your consciousness. By joining the tips of the thumb and index finger, for example, the internal energy cycles are completed, preventing dissipation.

You can also turn your palms upwards, with the index finger bowing down to the root of the thumb: this signifies the individual spirit (Jivatman) surrendering to the universal (Paratman). Another gesture is simply to sit with your hands cupped before you, palms turned upwards in order that you can receive the blessings of the universe.

Womb mudra

This is a most appropriate mudra for pregnancy. It binds the internal meridians to form a cohesive experience of inner security and harmony. To do this mudra, interlock the fingers of both hands, straightening your index fingers and thumbs against one another, and stretching your thumbs downwards. This creates the shape of your womb, the centre of your universe. You can use it during the early stages of labour. If you sit astride a chair and lean against its back, padded by a cushion, you can press the womb-shaped opening to your forehead. This helps you focus on the spiritual aspect of your opening womb.

Neti

Nasal congestion is common during pregnancy, due to the action of hormones on the mucous membranes. An effective way to bring relief is through Neti, an ancient cleansing practice in which you irrigate the nostrils with salt water. This cleanses the nose, resulting in easier breathing, greater resistance to bacteria, an enhanced sense of smell and increased mental clarity. Neti will also help with sinus problems, but don't do it if your sinuses are very congested. If you do Neti before your yoga practice it will enhance your breath awareness.

You can buy specially designed Neti pots, or use a small tea-pot with a smooth spout and a rounded lip. Add a teaspoonful of seasalt to a litre of boiled water – the same ratio as in the body – and cool to blood heat. Do Neti over a sink, and make sure the spout fits snugly inside your nostril. Tilt your head to the opposite side of the nostril you are doing, and relax, breathing through your mouth. Let the saline solution flow into one nostril and out of the other, into the sink. Pour an equal amount through both nostrils and then gently blow your nose, one nostril at a time. If your nose feels dry as a result, add a drop of vegetable oil to the water.

Om: the universal sound

Expelling the breath and making a sound at the same time helps release tension caused by negative thoughts and emotions. It is an excellent means of expressing yourself as you turn yourself inside out, both literally and metaphorically, during the process of giving birth. If you practise making sounds while pregnant, you will be less inhibited when you are in labour. It may seem odd to do this at first, but after some time you may notice how your experience changes. Using a simple mantra such as Om is a liberating experience, purifying both the self and the atmosphere.

Make sure you are in a safe and comfortable environment for this exercise. If you feel inhibited, your throat will close up.

'Om' is really 'Aum': 'a' as in 'cat', 'u' as in 'lurk' and 'm' as in 'hum'. Separate, they each perform a different function; together, they form the simple sound Om, in which the sum is greater than the parts.

The 'a' sound relates to the external world: we can improve our connection between the inner and outer states by making this sound. Start out softly and, as you make it, feel your whole abdominal area opening up. Aspirate from your belly, from your baby's cradle, and feel the sound getting louder. Do this as much as you like, to activate the Manipura chakra, the area of self-expression. It will centre you and bestow confidence and self-empowerment.

The 'u' sound relates to balance and equanimity. Make a long and steady 'uh' sound from the centre of your throat as you slowly turn your head from side to side in a sitting position. This activates Vishuddhi Chakra, the throat chakra, whose realm of influence is in communications. Be aware of your throat as the place of transition between the outer and inner worlds, and focus on clarity. Clear and appropriate communication leads to harmony.

The 'm' or 'mmmmm' sound relates to the internal world. The practice of bee (Bhramari) breath (see page 108) creates the reverberation of the 'mmmmmmm' sound in the head, just as the notes reverberate inside the gourd of a sitar. The result is a deeply calm and satisfying state of inner integrity.

By saying all three together in the mantra 'Om', we tune into the sound of the universe. Harmony arises, within and without. If you practise Om, in its parts and its whole, while you are pregnant, you open up yourself and your baby to the transformative experience of vibration at any time. Making sounds is a natural mechanism for releasing tension and pain on a deep level, and so making noises – any noises – during labour will help you accept and surrender to the contractions without inhibition.

CHAPTER FIVE

Yoga for the third trimester

During the third trimester of pregnancy you have the opportunity to feel more grounded than ever before, as you focus increasingly on the baby. This is the precious interface between potential and actuality, the 'dream-time' in which your accumulated prana, or Ojas, is transmitted to your child. As a result you will find that your approach to yoga becomes more and more meditative.

Continue to do yoga as described for the second trimester in chapter 4 but, as your posture, breathing and energy levels will all be changing, don't do any asana that now causes discomfort. Modify your stance, widening your legs in forward bends and using support when you can.

Avoid standing for long periods of time. Not only is this uncomfortable, but the uterus acts as a stop to the blood return from the legs, just as it would in a supine position. This can easily cause or aggravate haemorrhoids and varicose veins. To counteract this, do poses where the feet are higher than the heart, such as lying on your back with the legs up against a wall. To allow free pelvic circulation, place your buttocks 18 inches from the wall, or raise them on a cushion – or both.

As your pubic joint softens in preparation for widening during the birth, wide stances become less easy. With support, however, they may be very comfortable. All hip openers broaden the pelvis, improve the blood supply, relax the muscles and flush out energy blocks in preparation for labour day. Hip openers will relieve mild aching, but where there is disfunction, causing pain, kneeling positions are better.

In the last month or so, go more slowly than ever, concentrating on breathing, visualization or meditation, and relaxation. Use more cushions to prop yourself up and support the lower back. Alternate nostril breathing and bee breath are helpful in overcoming insomnia, and you can take advantage of the situation by meditating on your baby and visualizing a positive birth experience (see page 119).

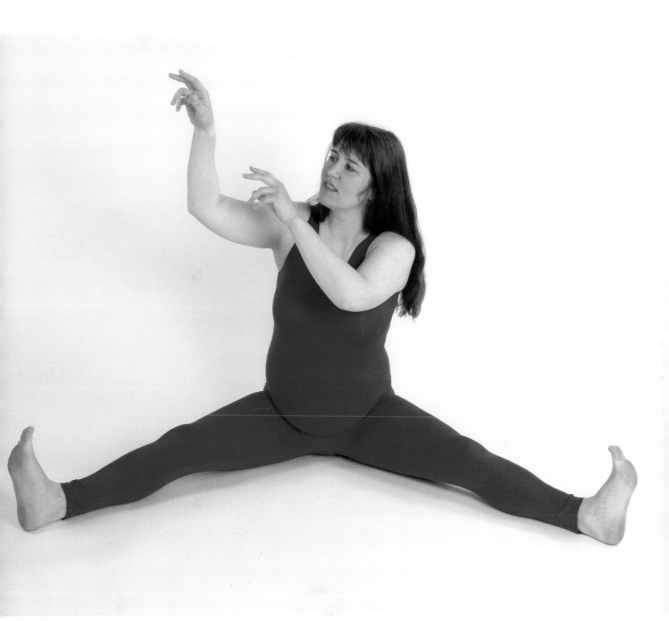

Ripe pomegranate

Among the Moslems of northwest China, the pomegranate is the symbol of fertility. During the last trimester, and especially the final month, your mood will naturally become more introspective as you prepare for your baby to emerge from the womb and a new life to begin. You will feel calm and yet at the same time expectant, as you anticipate the life-changing event of giving birth. You are a ripe pomegranate, replete with a mysterious inner abundance, ready to pop.

1 Supine against a wall

See page 62, but note that, to allow free pelvic circulation, you now should have your buttocks 18 inches away from the wall, or raised on a cushion – or both.

Caution: Omit this pose if it compresses your lungs. Instead, lie back with support under your back, shoulders and head.

2 The Cat
See page 56.

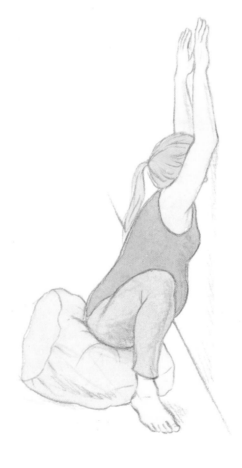

3 Squat

See also pages 57 and 63. You will probably have to sit on a stool or other support at this stage. You can stretch the shoulders at the same time by leaning against a wall.

Do Mula Bandha (see page 79) on the exhalation and release on the inhalation. Mula Bandha is more difficult in this position, but when you release you will experience how the muscles of your vagina will fold back when you are in labour. Repeat four or five times.

4 Tree prayer

Stand in the Mountain (page 53), resting one foot on a chair seat, toes turned out. Place your hands in the prayer position and gaze at your fingertips, relaxing the shoulders and focusing inwards.

Hold for as long as is comfortable. Repeat on the other side.

5 The Tree

See page 78. If raising the arms is now uncomfortable, adapt the pose by bending your arms over your head.

6 The Triangle

See page 54. For extra support, rest one hand on a chair.

7 Still summit

Go into the seated Mountain pose (page 66), but if your arms tingle when you raise them above your head, fold them as shown.

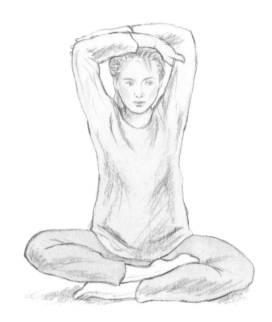

8 Waves of the Sea

Go into a seated angle pose (page 58). Think of your baby, enclosed in the little inland sea of your womb, the water against her skin in her microcosm: this is the sea, you are her earth.

With an upright back, raise your arms in front of you, hands at about eye level, and turn to your right.

Breathing easily, make a slight hissing sound with your tongue and teeth, like the sea, as you 'make waves' with your hands in the air, turning slowly to the left as you do so. Still waving your hands, return to face the front and go back the other way. Repeat this movement several times, and for as long as you like.

Visualize the easy grace of waves on the shoreline and feel the integration of earth and sea.

9 Child's pose

See page 58, but now do this pose over a beanbag or a pile of pillows.

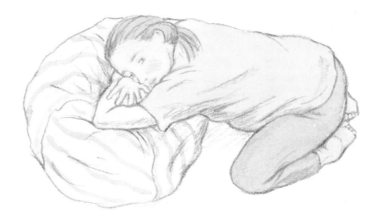

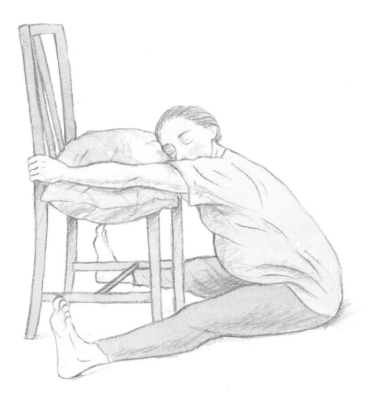

10 Seated angle pose

See page 58, but to create more room in the upper abdomen come forward on to a beanbag or chair rather than the floor.

11 Visualization

Do one of the visualization exercises described on the following pages. Alternatively, this is a good time to meditate (see page 120).

Positive visualizations

Pain in labour has less to do with the 'pain threshold' than fear of the unknown. Modern 'civilization' has separated us from the metaphysical nature of birth; information often comes from health care professionals rather than from our mothers or from witnessing others giving birth.

Yoga philosophy attributes difficulties encountered at any stage of life to be the outcome of karma, the idea that 'you reap what you sow', but this is not to say that we are helpless victims of destiny. We have freedom of choice, and can always activate Manipura chakra, empower ourselves, change our own karma and the world about us.

Inner balance creates the security we need to take responsibility for ourselves. A simple and effective way of implementing change on a deep level is to access the subconscious through visualization. If we treat ourselves with compassion and understanding, it becomes easier to change what we can – and to accept what we cannot.

The unbroken line: a linking exercise

Navel-gazing is a cliché of yoga but, like all clichés, it holds a ring of truth. You will notice that, as your pregnancy progresses, your navel protrudes; this exercise takes advantage of the fact that something usually so recessed is now so obvious. This simple yet powerful meditation helps us put our position as a mother in perspective. By doing it, we open ourselves up to a wider view, which engenders forgiveness, trust and courage.

Sit or lie comfortably so that you can place your right hand, palm taut, over your navel. Hold your left palm to the side and upwards, drawing down the grace of heaven.

Focus on your navel. Remember that once you were joined to your own mother by an umbilical cord, and that she nurtured you and gave you life when you too were a baby in her womb.

Take your mind to your mother's navel, and think of your grandmother: she gave your mother life, who gave you life. Your mother too was once as vulnerable as the child (her grandchild) you now carry in your womb.

Think of your grandmother's navel, and how she was once attached by an umbilical cord to your great-grandmother.

Think back to your great-grandmother's navel: she too had a mother, to whom she was once attached by an umbilical cord. And she too had a mother …

Trace the unbroken lineage, passed from mother to daughter via the umbilical cord, through the centuries. You will reach a point where you feel you are in a hall of mirrors, peeping into infinity. At this point, acknowledge the interface with eternity and listen to your own heartbeat. Feel yourself dissolving into awareness of the living chain, and retrace the trail back to the present.

Concentrate on the child attached by an umbilical cord to you now in your womb. Rejoice in your rich inheritance of wordless maternal love, and pass it on to your own child.

Visualizing the birth

One very effective tool for changing expectations is to make a tape with your own voice, in which you visualize a straightforward birth. Even if the birth is not as straightforward as you visualize it to be, the tape will boost your self-reliance before and during the birth. To make the tape, ensure that you are comfortable and won't be disturbed. Read the following suggested text out loud, slowly and clearly. Where there is an asterisk, leave a space of 20 to 30 seconds.

Lie in the Corpse pose, focusing on your breath. Breathe easily and softly. * As you breathe in, visualize a galaxy of tiny stars entering your lungs. * Watch them sparkling and shining as they quietly spread throughout your body. * Feel the light flooding right down to the tips of your toes. * Focus on your in-breath again, and feel the stars dancing up through your shoulders, down your arms, to the tips of your fingers. * Watch your breath, again turning into a Milky Way of stars, flowing up through your throat and into your head. * Watch the light, gently sweeping away every thought from your head. * As you breathe out, exhale any thoughts. * You feel very relaxed, and nothing is more important than this moment of complete release.**

Now take your mind down to your baby, and put yourself in his or her place: fastened secure-ly to you by the umbilical cord, your baby floats in the warm amniotic sea of the womb-world. Tumbling about like a baby dolphin in the earli-er months, stretching and snuggling in the later ones, she or he is completely aquatic. Your baby drinks and excretes the water, and the water cushions every movement. She or he can feel your heartbeat and sense your moods. For now, you are wrapped in the same aura; but one day it will be time for your baby to move on.*

At the bottom of your womb, where you know your cervix to be, envisage the closed bud of a lily flower floating on the surface of a still pond. It is sunrise on a clear morning; your baby has decided that it is too cramped in the womb, and has signalled to your body that it is time to open up. As the sun rises, watch the deep pink lily petals gradually unfolding, one by one, in its warmth. Each contraction comes to you as gently as the unfolding of the petals. Watch them carefully; concentrate on their individual beauty, on the way the sun illuminates them. They have their own rhythm and are aligned with the deep pulse of nature: watch them, trust them, go with them.* By the time the sun has risen, all the petals will be open, and your baby is ready to descend through the birth canal to meet you.

Feel the gentle pressure from your baby's head. It seems a tight fit, but the baby is able, by deep-rooted instinct, to get it just right. Visualize the joints of your pelvis expanding, feel your whole pelvic floor relaxing and giving; observe the ligaments and muscles folding back as your baby makes her way steadily through. Listen to your body's desire to push and go with it, breathing deeply and easily into the descent when the desire comes – and holding off when you need to gather strength for the next con-traction. Go with your baby, sending him or her courage, light and love.

Soon – not too fast and not too slowly, but in his or her own time – your baby is born, healthy, happy and unique. Rejoice in the miracle of new life as you bring your baby to your breast and you make eye contact for the first time.* Feel the warmth of the risen sun shining brightly on you both. * A new day begins. *

Now bring your mind back to the present, with your baby still tucked up snug and safe in your womb. Take a deep breath and exhale slowly, at length. * Focus on your breath for a couple of minutes before coming up, very slowly.

Meditation

Pregnancy can enhance sensitivity, awareness, self-knowledge and intu-ition, all of which are developed through yoga to become valuable tools in preparing for meditation. When choosing a meditation technique, use one of the greatest gifts of pregnancy yoga: your intuition. The decreased mobility and natural introspection of the latter months of pregnancy can be turned to advantage by the practice of meditation: the individual self becomes absorbed with the universal, and the sound-less rhythm of the cosmos becomes apparent.

J. Krishnamurti says: 'Meditation is the breeze that comes in when you leave the window open'. This book is about opening the window; it is only when you have forgotten that the window is open that the breeze appears. Meditation is a fruit that develops as a result of all the other practices described in this book: for example, asanas can be med-itation, gazing at a candle and positive visualization become meditation when self-consciousness is lost, and breath control is also a form of meditation. Specific techniques for meditation are not always necessary, since you can find them within all the other practices of yoga.

There are thousands of different meditation techniques, on which countless books have been written, but it is important to find one that suits you. A simple method recommended for beginners is to focus on an object or thought dear to you. Your baby is the perfect choice. This may not produce meditation *per se*, but forms a vital part of cultivating the necessary sense withdrawal, without which there can be no medita-tion. You can prepare for meditation with the following, all of which are to be found within this book:

- strengthening the body through asanas in order to sit comfortably to meditate
- balancing the subtle body with Pranayama
- developing relaxed concentration through Tratak (candle gazing)
- using mantra and visualization to focus and calm the thought waves

The transcendental experience of more subtle meditation is not some-thing to be learnt, but a state of grace that arises through a sincere atti-tude and synchronocity of circumstance. We have to drop all sense of ambition and ego, and the moment we think: 'I am meditating', it ceas-es to be. Above all, remember that meditation is the most natural state in the world. Clutch at it, and it will evaporate. Cease to strive for it, and you will be showered with indescribable gifts.

Part three

Labour, birth and afterwards

'You are the bows from which your children
as living arrows are sent forth.
The Archer sees the mark upon the path of
the infinite, and He bends you with His
might that His arrows may go swift and far.
Let your bending in the Archer's hand be
for gladness;
For even as He loves the arrow that flies, so
He loves also the bow that is stable.'

Kahlil Gibran, *The Prophet*

CHAPTER SIX

Labour and birth

Giving birth is a deeply instinctive process in which we can make further contact with the inner strength and space we have already found through yoga. A private, secure and comfortable environment provides the perfect cocoon for a relaxed labour, which will proceed more quickly (and therefore with fewer complications) as a result.

While some women prefer to give birth in hospital, for others a home birth in familiar surroundings is the ideal. However, life does not always work out as we plan it, and if certain situations occur you may be advised to give birth in hospital. Some of these may be problems that have been identified early in the pregnancy – for example thrombosis, low or high blood pressure, or an unusual blood group – or they may appear at the last minute. For example, if your waters have broken and more than 24 hours have elapsed without labour starting, there is an increased risk of uterine infection. If your pregnancy goes a fortnight past its due date, or the baby is breech, your midwives will also advise you to go to hospital.

When you are in labour, you release a hormone called oxytocin, which stimulates contractions. Adrenaline (epinephrine), secreted when we feel anxious and insecure, inhibits its production. An unknown environment with strangers present is thus likely to inhibit labour, and many women report that their contractions cease for a time after arriving in hospital. (The medical answer may be to put up a drip of synthetic oxytocin; thus is the doorway to further intervention opened.)

We have to be aware that certain situations may inhibit our instinctive reflexes, and sort them out while we can. This chapter outlines the important factors to consider before you go into labour, so that when the time comes you can be fully involved in the intensity of your internal experience without worrying about external distractions. Nobody else will know exactly how you feel when you are in labour, so you mustn't be afraid to voice your concerns.

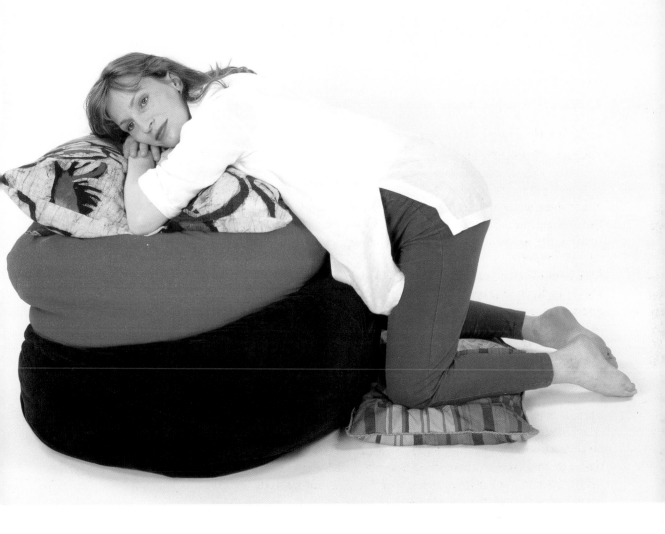

Creating the place of birth

Yoga helps you develop your flexibility and sensitivity. As your pregnancy advances and your preferences become clearer, you may change your mind about where you would like to give birth. If you find yourself giving birth in hospital when you had dreamed of doing so at home (or vice versa), you may feel disappointed, but it is kinder to yourself not to be too determined about where the birth is going to take place. The important thing is to be somewhere where you feel safe and secure, with supportive people around you and a midwife with whom you have shared your hopes and plans for the birth. The place of birth should afford privacy and calm, where you can listen to your body with the minimum of distractions.

At home, it is easy to create a relaxed atmosphere, but even if you are in hospital you can create your own environment, especially if you are in a room of your own. Having your own things with you, such as a yoga mat, low stool, beanbag or cushions, will help you feel more at home. You can take a portable music player, and use aromatherapy oils such as lavender (which is calming) or jasmine (which is enlivening). Bright lights in the room can be dimmed. You may not notice these things on a conscious level, but they will reinforce your sense of security and self-confidence.

The midwife

The French word for 'midwife' is 'sage-femme', meaning wise woman. Most midwives are very wise, and will tune into a labouring woman's mood and feelings as well as being on the alert for anything out of the ordinary. However, midwives are only human, and while many are wonderfully skilled and intuitive, others may be less sensitive. Birthing is an unpredictable process and, especially during a first labour, fear of the unknown may make a midwife's words seem more important than your own feelings. If conflict arises the stress it causes may, in the first stage of your labour, inhibit contractions.

If you have your own ideas but find you dare not voice them, you may find yourself outwardly going along with what the midwife tells you to do, but turn in upon yourself the pain of being unable to articulate a negative experience. Postnatal depression is often the outcome of a labour that has been technically well managed but emotionally mishandled. It is therefore extremely important to claim your right to a sensitive wise woman. If you go to hospital and find yourself attended by a midwife whom you find unsympathetic, then it is your right to ask for another.

A trusty companion
During labour, you will probably reach a stage when you are so absorbed in your bodily sensations that you cannot articulate your needs any longer. It is therefore important to be accompanied by someone who can speak for you when you have lost your voice. Your partner, your mother, sister or a friend who knows you and with whom you feel safe is invaluable. Go over your birthing plan with them beforehand and make sure that they know how you feel on every point. Be very clear and do not make any assumptions.

The stages of labour

Having made provision for your own protection as described, you can get on with the heart of the matter: giving birth to your baby. Once you are in labour, be prepared to drop linear thought and turn your attention inward. Birthing is a very powerful and primitive process, and instinct will dictate to you what positions are suitable. By having practised yoga while pregnant, your body is pre-programmed to the possibilities. Your intuition, which is in any case particularly strong during pregnancy and childbirth, will tell you what you need to do. Trust it.

Technically, labour takes place in three stages. The first stage consists of contractions of the uterus as the neck of the cervix opens up; the second stage is when the baby makes its descent down the birth canal; the third stage is the delivery of the placenta. Between the first and second stages comes a period known as 'transition'. Each of these stages is different and has different requirements.

The first stage

During the first stage, the uterus tips forward in the abdomen and the contractions open the cervix. This opening is measured in centimetres, and when you are 'ten centimetres dilated' your cervix is fully open and the baby is ready to make its descent down the birth canal.

The way the cervix opens up to these ten centimetres can vary enormously from woman to woman: it may take hours or even days; it can be painful or painless. Your experience of menstrual periods is a guide to what to expect: if you have painful periods you will generally experience more discomfort in the first stage than if you have pain-free ones. For most women, the contractions feel at first like period pains, which gradually become more intense.

In any case, the first stage of a first labour will probably be the longest, since this is the first time your body has done this. What you do in this stage depends on how long the process is taking. For example, though movement is recommended in labour, in the early stages you may wish to rest, or take a warm bath to relax you, conserving your energy for later. If your cervix is taking a long time to open, either walk around, sit in a supported squat, or go on all fours, step one foot forwards and rock gently (see the rocking lunge, page 72).

There is a connection between the mouth and the cervix – if your mouth is open, the cervix will likewise release. Practise doing aspirated 'Ohhh!'s and 'Ahhh!'s in a kneeling position while reaching up with your arms, as shown on page 49. As you progress through this stage, become uninhibited about making louder sounds.

Visualization in the first stage of labour

Although the word 'contraction' is unfortunately associated with tightness, if you think of contractions rather as 'openings', you will soften from within. Try to focus on the opening of the cervix and visualize it as the unfolding of lotus petals. Breathe into the openings and see each one as a release. Articulating this release with womanly hollering will help open you up from within and lighten your whole being. Though it may sound like wails of pain from the outside, your inner experience will be of glorious expansion. Do not be inhibited, and even if it does feel like pain and the term 'glorious expansion' seems absurd, keep taking your attention back to the opening of your inner flower.

If you use a mantra or a prayer, visualize it emanating from the heart of the lotus. Stay with your inner focus and do not be swayed by external considerations – they have all been taken care of now. Express yourself when you need to, but avoid conversation.

During the birthing process, nature supplies us with extra endorphins, hormones that act as a natural pain relief. Many women speak of going to 'another planet', as they enter a trance-like state. Giving birth is perhaps the greatest meditation technique we will ever have: take it as a gift.

Water in labour

Immersion in water provides one of the most marvellous forms of pain relief. It not only buoys up your physical body, but also provides you with a safe and secure place in which you will find it easier to go with your instincts. Michel Odent, who pioneered water births in the 1970s, began by using a child's paddling pool, and many hospitals now provide special birthing pools.

Water can have a miraculous effect on the opening process: even the sound of running water causes some women to dilate so rapidly that they have given birth by the time the pool has filled. If you hire a pool for use at home, install it in good time so that you can build up an experience of the pool as 'your place'.

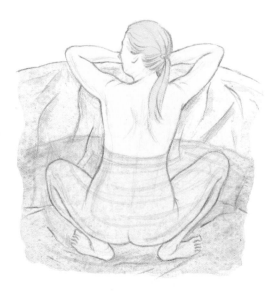

If you do not have a birthing pool, an ordinary bath, or even a shower, does fine. For many of the benefits of a birthing pool in shallow water, go on all fours and have someone pour water over your lower back.

Transition

When you are almost fully dilated you will find yourself 'in transition' between the first and second stages. Your baby's head is positioned against the open cervix, usually facing your sacrum, and you will be flooded with the hormone adrenaline (epinephrine), which will prepare your body for the huge effort required of you. The expulsive reflex of the second stage begins to take over from the contractions of the first, and you will feel suddenly recalled from your 'other planet'. This can be an emotional experience: you may feel fearful, sick, or have a great desire to drink. Sucking a natural sponge soaked with water can be welcome. Transition may take anything from a few minutes to a few hours.

The second stage

The second stage begins when you find yourself overtaken again by internal impulses – this time by an overwhelming desire to push or bear down. This process, when the uterus expels the baby and forces its descent, may take minutes or hours, and will probably be slower with the first baby than subsequent ones.

If you have been resting, you may wish to change position now; make sure that the position you adopt does not inhibit the opening of your coccyx. The semi-reclining position is much less efficient than positions that enlist the help of gravity, such as a supported squat, being on all fours, or a supported standing position. If you are on a bed, you can always turn around and, in a kneeling position, hold on to the back of the bed. If you are tired and lying down, lie on your side so that nothing inhibits the opening of the pelvis.

The baby's skull is soft and made of plates that overlap to form a point that helps its descent. As she moves down the birth canal, she will slowly rotate her head until it 'crowns' – becomes visible – at the entrance to the vagina. At this point you may release a primal cry as you surrender to the spontaneous action of your body. Your midwife can assist you through the final contractions, when the head, then the shoulders, and the rest of the baby are born.

The third stage

In modern obstetrics it is common to use an injection of a drug to help the placenta out. Unless the placenta is stuck, however, this is unnecessary. The quickest and most natural way of expelling the placenta is to sit upright after the birth and suckle your baby as soon as possible. Given 20 or 30 minutes, or up to an hour, the placenta will come out all in one piece and of its own accord (a cough will help it on its way).

Positions for labour

Every labour is different. Practise the following positions beforehand, in order to help your body remember what to do naturally when you are in labour. During the labour itself, tune into your instincts: if you try one position and find it uncomfortable, leave it; if your body chooses something unheard of, never mind: it is the position for you.

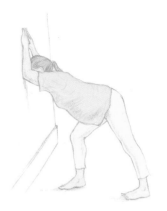

Kneeling

Kneeling with knees apart and resting on a beanbag or pile of cushions (right) is a grounding position, especially in the late first stage.

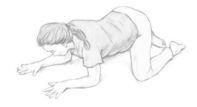

Upright

The more upright you are, the more you are using one of nature's greatest gifts – gravity. During the first stage, simply walking around and keeping mobile can help you progress, but take care not to become too tired. Squatting is ideal, but it may be difficult to sustain without support. Squatting on a low stool is a good position.

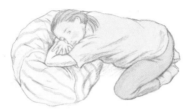

All fours

If upright positions are tiring, or the contractions are too fast or overwhelming, an all-fours position is useful. Put cushions under your knees (sore knees can persist for days after the birth). Alternatively, kneel and lean forwards over a beanbag or a chair (see page 123) – any position is better than sitting on your tailbone.

If the baby is descending too fast, go down into the Sphinx (above) with your chest and arms on the floor and put your bottom in the air. 'Panting' with your mouth open will also inhibit the bearing-down process.

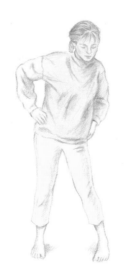

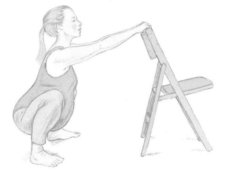

Alternatively, your partner could support you from behind or in front, or you could hold on to the back of a chair (above) with a cushion under your heels. You could stand leaning against your birth companion or lunge against a wall (top). If you feel too tired to stand upright, try standing and leaning against the bed. Hip circles (left) are also helpful. Use your body in whatever way comes naturally.

Checklist for labour

When you are in labour you may find it difficult to think in the normal linear way. Don't fight it – this is nature's way of helping you deal instinctively with the powerful, primitive initiation process of birthing. Have this list available for your companions to remind you of what you might do. If you have low back pain, ask a companion to soothe it with a gentle massage, or simply have something warm there, such as a lavender and wheat pillow.

The first stage

• Try to keep mobile and upright as much as possible, but don't wear yourself out.

• Do hip circles, keep walking.

• Wall-lunges and supported squatting are useful.

• Place cushions under your knees when they are on the floor.

• Do the rocking lunge gently backwards and forwards, to help open up the cervix.

• There is a connection between the mouth and the cervix – if your mouth is open and you are uninhibited in making sounds, the cervix will likewise release. At the same time try reaching up with your arms.

• If your labour is long, remember to empty your bladder regularly.

• Breathe slowly and evenly into the centre of your being.

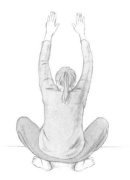

Transition

• At this stage you will probably feel tired and thirsty; take small sips of water or suck on a wet sponge.

• If transition is prolonged because the anterior lip of the cervix is slow to withdraw over the baby's head, go into the Sphinx.

• If the urge to push is strong, but your midwife tells you not to push yet, it helps to blow out firmly instead, as if blowing out a candle.

The second stage

• Don't be inhibited about crying 'Ohhh!' and 'Ahhh!' as you 'bear down' with the muscles of the pelvic floor. You can do this standing or kneeling.

• Leaning forward over a chair or other support will help to free and open the whole pelvic region.

• A supported squat opens up the birth canal and utilizes gravity.

• If you want to slow down the contractions, do a Sphinx.

• Breathe into the centre of your being, and all will be well.

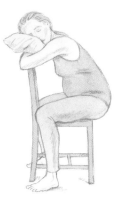

CHAPTER SEVEN

Life after birth

The change from being pregnant to having a baby to care for is enormous: whereas in the last trimester of pregnancy the body's energies are drawn inward, the breakthrough of labour brings with it a new, outward focus. A period of rest and adjustment is vital for you both, as you become attuned to your new life together.

Your newborn baby now has a face, a name and a character to discover. Your mood, however, may still be introverted as you reflect on the momentous events of the birth and adjust to your new separateness from your baby and your new life as a mother. Birthing is nature's initiation ceremony. In becoming a mother, a woman is claiming her birthright and realizing her independence, sometimes for the first time.

While it is important to rest after giving birth, too much rest can slow the circulation and delay healing. Some exercises can be introduced from the first day, and you can gradually build on them over the coming days, weeks and months. With all the focus on the baby, it is easy to forget about your own well-being. As you are the fount of your baby's health you should also nurture yourself. One of the best ways of doing this is through yoga.

People's approach to postpartum yoga can vary enormously, and much depends on your individual birth experience and your interpretation of what yoga is. You may want to resume your yoga practice immediately, or wait six weeks before doing any, or build up slowly and gradually over a few months. Recognize your individual needs before doing any exercise more taxing than toe wiggles, and be easy on yourself during the postpartum period. Try not to spend too much time on your feet, and avoid lifting anything heavy. Roll in and out of bed, using your arms to assist your abdominal muscles, and if you squat (for example to attend to a toddler) support the pelvic floor by sitting on a low stool or beanbag. Nonetheless, any yoga, at any level, will bring great benefits to you, your baby and the whole family.

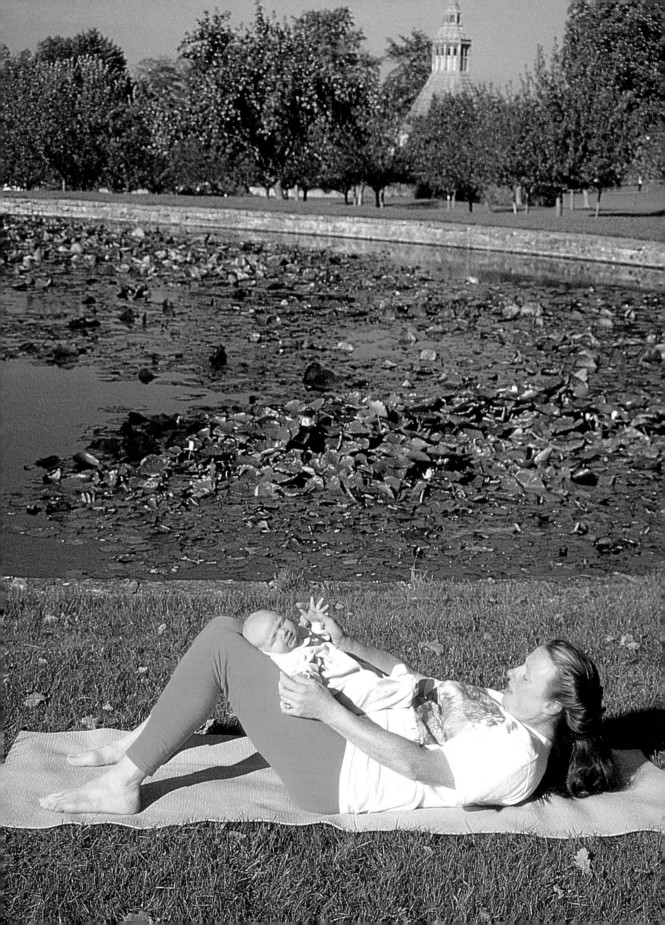

The mind and body after childbirth

As soon as the baby is born and the placenta is out, your body begins to close up again. Changes in hormonal production cause the joints in the pelvic girdle to firm up and the milk to flow. Breastfeeding in turn stimulates involution – that is, the womb retracts back to its pre-pregnancy size, simultaneously shedding its residual pregnancy lining in a flow of blood known as lochia. This process takes about six weeks in all. During the first few days you may experience pain in the uterus as it contracts during breastfeeding, especially with a second or third baby, but it soon passes. The pain-relieving qualities of water are not restricted to birthing, so take warm baths when you can. If you have a birthing pool you can feed your baby in the water.

Increased activity and standing up will stimulate the flow of lochia, and rest will reduce it. Since the cervix is still somewhat open from the birth, do not exert pressure on the pelvic floor, which may lead to a risk of a prolapsed uterus (when it drops down into the vagina). Treat the whole pelvic area, however quick and easy the birth, with respect.

Breastfeeding

Breast milk is the best food for your baby, and will give him or her the best possible start for a healthy life. It can also bring great joy and pleasure to you as a mother, but is not always as simple to do as it looks. Although breastfeeding can be an important way to bond with your baby, breastfeeding problems can be the quickest and easiest way to stress. Find out as much as you can about breastfeeding before your baby is born.

Many babies suckle soon after birth, but not all. As breastfeeding anxiety can be counterproductive, ensure that you have as calm and peaceful an environment as possible in which to feed your new baby. If you both feel safe and relaxed, breastfeeding will be easier. Breastfeeding in itself stimulates the relaxation response.

Sometime on the second or third day after the birth your milk will 'come in', that is, the initial thick and creamy colostrum becomes more watery and copious. Your breasts may become engorged with milk, which makes them feel hard and uncomfortable for a day or two. Feed your baby frequently until the demand catches up with the supply, and take warm baths or place hot flannels over the breasts to relieve discomfort.

The milk coming in may bring the third-day 'blues', a temporary feeling of depression or weepiness. It may seem strange, even shocking, to feel so low if you have been feeling elated, but it is a natural response to changing hormone levels and the new physical demands being placed upon you. The best way to deal with third-day blues is to accept them as a natural process that will soon pass. Do not have too many expectations of yourself and get as much help with housework and other tasks as you can, so that you can live in rhythm with your baby. When you feel low, practise breathing and relaxation techniques, meditate, or simply try and detach yourself by listening to relaxing music and counting your blessings.

The subtle body

Labour is hard work. Even the smoothest, easiest labour uses up enormous quantities of the body's apana, or downward-moving prana. Added to this is the fact that during the last four weeks of your pregnancy you have been bestowing your accumulated prana on your baby in the form of Ojas. Moreover, as the apana continues to dominate for the first six weeks postpartum, you will feel depleted in prana. The slightest activity, such as making a cup of coffee, may be a challenge.

Mothers often feel as if they are 'brain-dead' when they have just given birth, but this feeling may be seen as a great gift: 'our brains are removed that our hearts might hear'. Patanjali says, in his second sutra, 'Yoga is the cessation of the fluctuations of mind-stuff'. 'Brain-dead' becomes what the sages of old called the gift of Unity Consciousness, where we lose our focus on the small picture only to gain an experience of the larger one. New mothers with their suckling infants might feel themselves to be – perhaps for the first time – a vital component of nature, one harmonious note in the universal Om.

Bonding with your baby

Our understanding of our new place in the world as mothers is instinctive, not intellectual. These first moments, days, weeks and even months of cuddling, gazing, kissing and nourishing assure a firm connection between mother and child. This bonding is an important part of an emotional process that, if repressed, may result in postnatal depression for you, and feelings of alienation and emotional bereavement for the child in later life.

In today's fast-paced society it is considered usual to have many visitors and to return to normal activities as soon as possible. Although it is exciting to show off a new baby, rising to other people's expectations when you are trying to concentrate on breastfeeding and getting to know your child inevitably results in exhaustion and irritation. You need to recover your strength, and savour the precious early days with your baby that will never come again.

Yoga postpartum

Usually when we think of yoga we conjure up images of the asanas, but when you have just had a baby the definition of yoga expands to encompass everything that you do – or don't do. It is possible to begin gentle toning and stretching on the day you gave birth, but don't make any unrealistic demands on yourself.

Circulation
To keep the circulation lively while resting, sit on the edge of the bed or chair and rotate your ankles half a dozen times each way.

The pelvic floor
Pelvic-floor exercises (see page 46) can be done immediately, even if you have had stitches, since they help close the wound and speed healing. They may cause discomfort at first, and don't do them if you are already in pain. To help you remember to do them, use a trigger such as feeding time. The exercises are more interesting if done as Mula Bandha (page 79), and can be done in any position, including a pelvic tilt (below).

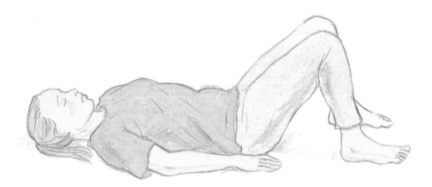

The back
When you have to lift things, bend your knees, draw your pelvic floor muscles up and your abdominals in, holding the object or child close to you. If you are lifting laterally, move your feet first rather than twisting at the waist. Stretch your back whenever you can.

The hips
Before the birth you tried to widen the pelvic joints; now you want to close them. Sit in a kneeling position rather than cross-legged and focus on closing exercises such as the Cow-head pose part 2 (page 93) and the Thunderbolt (page 59).

The shoulders

Breastfeeding and bending over a baby may cause aching shoulders. Place your baby on a pillow on your lap to feed her. Try not to hunch your shoulders, and support your back and have your feet flat on the floor, on a stool if necessary. Alternatively, feed your baby lying down, supporting your head and shoulders with pillows.

Whenever you sit down, ensure that your lower back is supported. Open up your shoulders whenever you can: arm extensions (page 42) or simply stretching up while deeply inhaling can feel wonderful. You can also clasp your hands behind your back and rotate your head any time. Kneeling close to a wall and leaning into it with your arms above your head is a delicious shoulder stretch (right), as is doing a standing forward bend against a table or work surface.

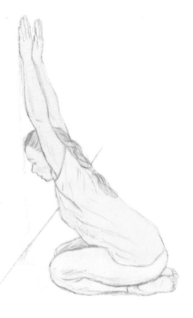

The abdominal muscles

The abdominal muscles may feel floppy and your abdomen enlarged for several weeks or even months postpartum. Start doing the following toning exercises, along with gentle twists (both supine and sitting) to help develop the transverse muscles. Strong abdominal muscles will support the back and reduce the risk of backache.

The pair of straight (rectus) muscles running down the front of your stomach may have separated during pregnancy. To check, lie on your back with your legs bent and your feet flat on the floor. Place your thumb a couple of inches above your navel, and, on an exhalation, slowly lift your head up to look at your knees (below). If you feel resistance against your thumb, your muscles are still together; if there is none, or if you feel the muscles constricting, then they have separated.

If this has happened, do pelvic cross-tilts regularly (see next page), and they will rejoin in time. Otherwise go on to supine pelvic tilts (page 67), straight after delivery if you wish. All tilts will help the uterus regain its original position, as well as toning the abdominal muscles.

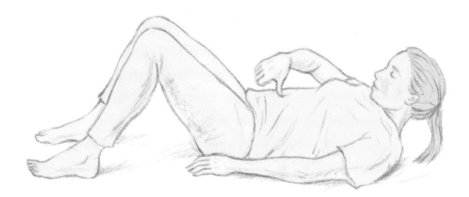

Pelvic cross-tilts

If you do about four batches of this exercise daily your rectus muscles will soon come back together. Do not rush the process, however, but let them come back in their own time.

Lie flat on your back with your knees bent, feet flat on the floor, hip-width apart, the ankles a few inches from the buttocks. This is the base position. Cross your arms over your abdomen so your right hand is over your left side and vice versa.

As you exhale, gently contract your abdominal muscles, breathing them down to your spine, and, simultaneously raising your head a couple of inches from the floor, hold your sides with your hands, so they create a gentle supportive corset. Draw your chin down to your sternum. Release back down on the inhalation. Repeat five times and relax. When you have done, gently roll your head from side to side.

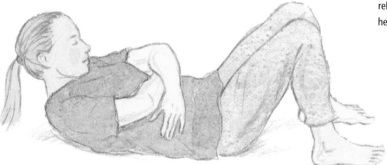

Pelvic curl-ups

Once you can do pelvic tilts easily, go one step further and curl up your abdomen.

Caution: If you have discomfort in your neck, do not raise your head or arms.

Assume the base position (see pelvic cross-tilts, above) and take your arms above your shoulders, bending your elbows so your palms face upwards.

Inhale, and as you exhale, draw your abdominal muscles down to your spine as for the pelvic tilt above. Draw up the muscles of your pelvic floor in Mula Bandha, simultaneously raising your head and crossing your arms so your hands touch the opposite thighs. As you raise your head, take the tension out of your jaw by tucking your chin down to your sternum.

As you inhale, slowly uncurl back to the floor. Relax as you inhale and repeat up to five times.

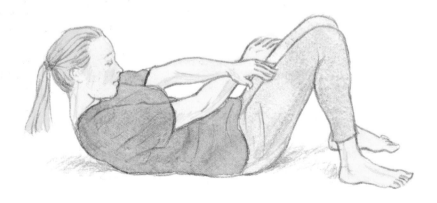

Crossover

Do this when you feel stronger, probably after about a fortnight. This strengthens the transverse abdominal muscles.

Lie on your back, as for pelvic tilts. Inhale, and on the exhalation, do Mula Bandha, flattening your lumbar spine to the floor.

Curl your head up and reach one hand across to the outside of the opposite thigh.

Inhale, release, and repeat on the other side. Repeat up to five times a side per session.

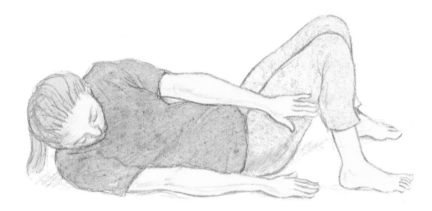

Yoga following a Caesarean

It is essential to have medical approval before practising yoga after a Caesarean, as there may be other factors to consider. Any abdominal exercises, and even shoulder openers that may stretch the abdomen, should be introduced very gently, preferably not until about six weeks.

You can still do pelvic-floor exercises, however. Even though the muscles of the pelvic floor are much less stressed than in a vaginal delivery, they have still borne the weight of pregnancy and need toning. And there's no reason not to rest, relax and do abdominal breathing and alternate nostril breathing.

Making time for yoga

Finding time to do yoga might seem too much effort in the beginning, but even a small amount will reward you with extra vitality and a feeling of being more in control of your time and situation. If at first you can't manage it, don't worry – let the yoga come to you. That is, don't see yoga as something separate from the rest of your life, but integrate it.

Be aware of your posture while looking after the baby, do pelvic lifts while lying in bed and pelvic-floor exercises any time. It's just a matter of getting into the habit. With regular practice, you will find it easier to set aside time for yoga. It is better and easier to do yoga for 10 to 15 minutes at a time several times a day than in one hour-long session.

Caution: Because the pelvic joints are now closing, any pose that widens the hips is undesirable during the first six weeks postpartum. Positions that put strain on the abdomen and back are also contra-indicated. Avoid the Warriors, the Triangle and the seated angle pose, don't stretch too far sideways, or overdo twists. Avoid full back bends until at least six months after the birth, and don't do forward bends until the milk supply has stabilized. Omit all inverted poses until the flow of lochia stops.

Yoga beyond the first six weeks

Test your body's readiness to return to more vigorous poses by jumping lightly up and down and coughing at the same time. If you leak urine, continue with pelvic-floor exercises until you can do it without leakage. You could cause problems in the future by stressing weak muscles at this point.

The Cobra

Once the initial six-week period is over, and when you begin to feel ready for slightly stronger abdominal exercises, begin with the Cobra.

Lie prone with your hands and forearms flat on the floor, elbows under your shoulders. Keeping your pubic bone on the floor (cushioned with a blanket if necessary), breathe in, opening up your sternum and lengthening your abdomen forwards, like a snake creeping along on its belly. As you exhale, sink your navel down towards the floor. Repeat three times and rest.

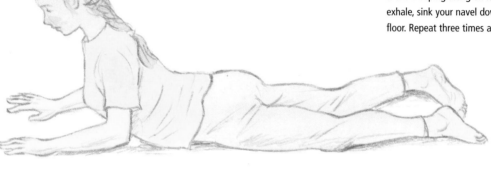

Now place your hands slightly in front of your shoulders, fingers spread. Come up on an inhalation, lengthening the whole spine forwards and up. Keep your shoulders down and your elbows tucked into your sides, slightly bent to avoid jamming your shoulders up.

Look ahead, opening the sternum as you inhale, lowering slightly as you exhale. Maintain for two or three breaths.

Counteract this movement by lying on your back with your knees bent up over your chest, and rock gently from side to side. Follow it with a gentle twist to release the lower back.

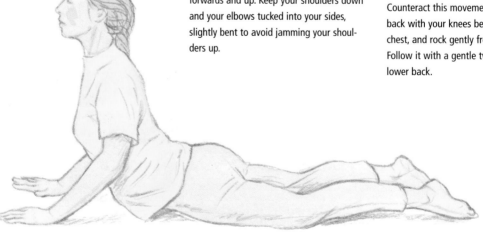

The Boat

This is a strong stomach exercise, so don't do it until you are ready for it. Neither should you attempt it if you have any weakness in the lower back. Start by doing it against a wall, and progress to the unsupported version.

Sit on the floor with your legs together and your hands by your sides. Bend your knees and lift your feet from the floor. Leaning back slightly, straighten your legs and balance them against the weight of your upper body.

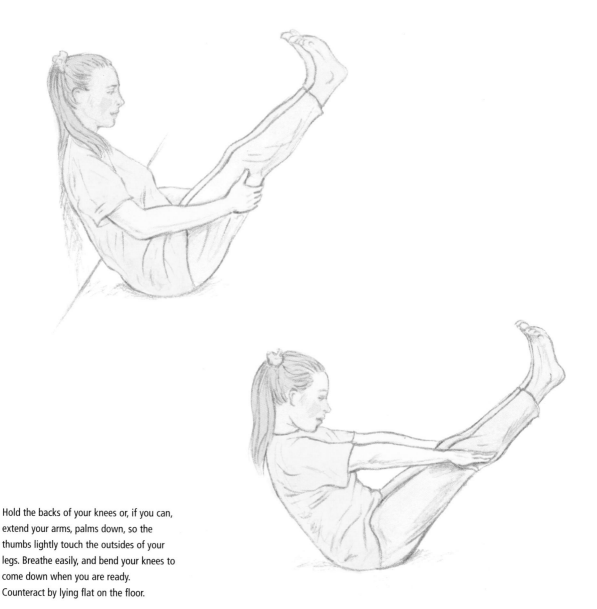

Hold the backs of your knees or, if you can, extend your arms, palms down, so the thumbs lightly touch the outsides of your legs. Breathe easily, and bend your knees to come down when you are ready. Counteract by lying flat on the floor.

Exercising with your baby

There are ways of integrating your baby into your exercise as she grows – she can be useful, and have fun too. You can sit her on your tummy as you do pelvic tilts and curls, lay her on the floor as you do your Cat pose over her or, as she grows, sit her on your knee as you do sitting forward bends. You can hug her to you as you roll from side to side and just let her join in your practice as she gains independence. Children are natural yogis.

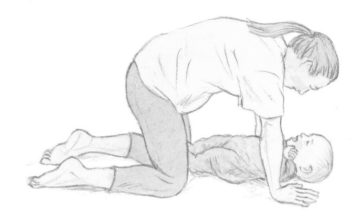

Pranayama, meditation and relaxation

Meditation with a new baby often occurs spontaneously. Young babies naturally tune into their mother's breathing patterns and even their brainwaves. You will probably find that your baby loves to lie on you, ear to your heart, and will fall asleep as you relax into the Corpse. As long as their mother is close by, babies rarely seem to cry during Pranayama or even deep meditation. If your baby is wakeful, arrange for someone else to look after her for an hour or so once a week.

Because of the turmoil of the transition from pregnancy to motherhood, emphasize calming rather than energizing breaths. Particularly useful is alternate nostril breathing (Nadi Sodhana), since it balances all the energies of the body and replaces confusion with harmony.

The yoga of food

Many new mothers expect to lose weight when they do yoga, especially if breastfeeding, and are disappointed when this does not happen. Reducing food intake, however, in a desire to lose weight is unhealthy during the postpartum period because it results in less milk for the baby and less energy for you. If you exercise the yoga of food with a varied and nutritious diet, eating enough to generate sufficient milk for the baby, you will eventually recover your figure. It is believed that the hormone prolactin, responsible for milk production, also causes water retention, so that the extra weight often disappears once the baby is weaned. While it is unrealistic to expect to lose weight quickly, a balanced diet and gentle yoga exercise will bring acceptable results in time. Yoga is not just a system of stretching and meditation: yoga is awareness, yoga is living in the present, yoga is union, synthesis and integrity. Yoga is life.

Further reading and useful addresses

Balaskas, Janet, *New Active Birth*, Thorsons, 1991

Balaskas, Janet *New Natural Pregnancy*, Gaia, 1998

Balaskas, Janet & Gordon, Yehudi, *Water Birth*, Thorsons, 1990

Balaskas, Janet & Gordon, Yehudi, *The Encyclopedia of Pregnancy and Birth*, Macdonald Orbis, 1987

Baldwin, Rahima & Richardson, Terra Palmarim, *Pregnant Feelings*, Celestial Arts (CA), 1986

Bourne, Gordon, *Pregnancy*, Pan, 1989

Chamberlain, David, *The Mind of Your Newborn Baby*, North Atlantic Books (Berkeley, CA), 1998

Chopra, Deepak, *Perfect Weight*, Rider Books, 1994

Easwaran, Eknath, *The Bhagavad Gita*, Penguin Arkana, 1986

Easwaran, Eknath, *The Upanishads*, Arkana, 1988

Fletcher, Gillian, *Get into Shape After Childbirth*, Ebury, 1991

Freedman, Francoise Barbira, & Hall, Doriel, *Yoga for Pregnancy*, Ward Lock, 1998

Gardner, Joy, *Healing Yourself During Pregnancy*, McNaughton & Gunn, Michigan 1987

Gibran, Kahlil *The Prophet*, Heinemann, 1926

Hughes, Helga, *The Complete Prenatal Water Workout Book*, Avery Publishing Group Inc., 1989

Huxley, Laura Archera & Ferrucci, Piero, *The Child of Your Dreams*, Destiny Books, Vermont, 1992

Isherwood, Christopher, & Swami Prabhavananda, *How to Know God*, Mentor Books, 1953

Kitzinger, Sheila, *The Complete Book of Pregnancy and Childbirth*, Penguin, 1999

Kitzinger, Sheila, *Homebirth and Other Alternatives to Hospital*, Dorling Kindersley, 1995

Lad, Dr Vasant *Ayurveda, The Science of Self-Healing*, Lotus Press, 1984

Lawrence Beech, Beverley, *Who's Having Your Baby?*, Bedford Square Press, 1991

Leboyer, F. *Birth Without Violence*, Cedar, 1995

Lim, Robin, *After The Baby's Birth ... A Woman's Way to Wellness*, Celestial Arts (CA), 1991

Mehta, Silva & Shyam, *Yoga the Iyengar Way*, Dorling Kindersley, 1990

O'Connor, Marie, *Birthtides*, Pandora/HarperCollins, 1995

Odent, Dr Michel, *Birth Reborn*, Souvenir, 1994

Odent, Dr Michel, *Entering the World*, Marion Boyars, 1984

Odent, Dr Michel, *The Nature of Birth and Breastfeeding*, Bergin and Garvey, 1992

Polden, Margie, & Whiteford, Barbara, *The Postnatal Exercise Book*, Frances Lincoln, 1992

Renfrew, Mary & Fisher, Chloe, & Arms, Suzanne, *Bestfeeding – Getting Breastfeeding Right for You*, Celestial Arts, (Berkeley, CA), 1990

Tiron, Denise & Mack, Sue, *Complementary Therapies for Pregnancy & Childbirth*, Balliere Tindall, 1995

Trungpa, Chogyam *Shambhala, The Sacred Path of the Warrior*, Shambhala Publications, 1984

Verney, Dr Thomas, with Kelly, John, *The Secret Life of the Unborn Child*, Warner Books, 1998

Wesson, Nicky, *Homebirth*, Vermilion

Wesson, Nicky, *Labour Pain*, Vermilion/Ebury, 1999

Association of Breastfeeding Mothers
26 Holmshaw Close, London SE26 4TH
Tel: 0208 778 4767

Association for Improvements in the Maternity Services (AIMS)
40, Kingswood Avenue, London NW6 6LS
Tel: 0208 960 5585

Caesarean Support Network
2, Hurst Park Drive, Huyton, Liverpool L36 1TF
Tel: 0151 480 1184

Independent Midwives Association
Nightingale Cottage, Shamblehurst Lane, Botley, Southampton SO32 2BY
Tel: 02380 694429

La Leche League
BM3424, London WC1N 3XX
Tel: 0207 242 1278

National Childbirth Trust
Alexandra House, Oldham Terrace, Acton, London W3 6NH
Tel: 0208 9928637

The Yoga Biomedical Trust, Yoga Therapy Centre Royal London Homeopathic Hospital Trust, 60 Great Ormond Street, London WC1N 3HR.
Tel: 0207 419 7195

Index

Note: **bold** figures indicate descriptions of poses and exercises

ACKNOWLEDGEMENTS

My warmest thanks to all my yoga teachers (especially BKS Iyengar, John Hawkins, Danielle Arin, Ruth White and Derek Thorne) for their inspiration; to all the midwives (especially Jenny Moss), doctors (especially Michel Odent) and physiotherapists who have shared their expertise; to all the pregnant women and mothers it has been my privilege to meet and talk to during the evolution of this book; to Angie Rooke and Jennie Thomas for modelling so patiently. I would like to acknowledge all the team at Gaia who helped put this together: thank you to Pip Morgan for rescuing the manuscript from the back of a drawer; to Sarah Theodosiou for disentangling cryptic Sanskrit into coherent page layouts; to Lucy Su for her delicate illustrations; and especially to Sarah Chapman for her consistent good humour and skilful editing. Finally I must thank my husband, Bradley, without whom none of this would have been possible, and our children for simply being.

OTHER TITLES PUBLISHED BY GAIA BOOKS LTD

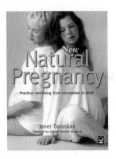

NEW NATURAL PREGNANCY
Janet Balaskas
£8.99
ISBN 1 85675 074 4

Diet, exercise and preparation for a healthy baby and a healthy you.

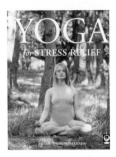

YOGA FOR STRESS RELIEF
Swami Shivapremananda
£11.99
ISBN 1 85675 028 0

Yoga positions, breathing exercises and meditation for the relief and prevention of stress symptoms.

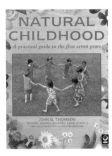

NATURAL CHILDHOOD
John B. Thomson et al
£18.99 hardback
£14.99 paperback
ISBN 1 85675 091 4 hardback
ISBN 1 85675 022 1 paperback

A new style of conscious parenting that helps parents make informed choices about play, health and education.

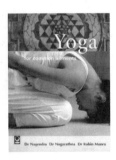

YOGA FOR COMMON AILMENTS
Dr Robin Monro,
Dr Nagarathna, Dr Nagendra
£8.99
ISBN 1 85675 010 8

Clear, simple exercises to counteract many conditions including stress, insomnia and heart disease.

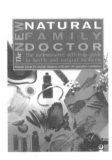

NEW NATURAL FAMILY DOCTOR
General Editor
Dr Andrew Stanway
£12.99
ISBN 1 85675 057 4

A comprehensive guide to choosing natural therapies to suit a particular ailment.

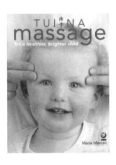

TUI NA MASSAGE
for a healthier, brighter child
Maria Mercati
£9.99
ISBN 1 85675 125 2

Gentle massage sequences to ease many babyhood and childhood ailments including teething, colic, fevers, bumps and bruises.

To request a catalogue or to order any of the titles above please call 01453 752985, fax 01453 752987 or e-mail info@gaiabooks.co.uk. Or you can write to us at 20 High Street, Stroud, Gloucestershire, GL5 1AZ. Have you seen our website? Go to: www.gaiabooks.co.uk